lighter

lighter

ELIMINATE EMOTIONAL EATING

Create Lasting

and Healthy Habits to

Lose Weight & Keep it

Off for Life Without

the Struggle

ERIKA FLINT

NEW YORK

LONDON • NASHVILLE • MELBOURNE • VANCOUVER

Lighter

Eliminate Emotional Eating: Create Lasting and Healthy Habits to Lose Weight & Keep It Off for Life Without the Struggle

Published in New York, New York, by Morgan James Publishing in partnership with Difference Press. Morgan James is a trademark of Morgan James, LLC. www.MorganJamesPublishing.com

The Morgan James Speakers Group can bring authors to your live event. For more information or to book an event visit The Morgan James Speakers Group at www. TheMorganJamesSpeakersGroup.com.

ISBN 9781683507789 PB
ISBN 9781683507796 EB

Library of Congress
Control Number: 2017914804

Front Cover Designer: Chris Treccani, 3 Dog Creative (www.3dogcreative.net)
Interior Design by: Glen Edelstein, Hudson Valley Book Design

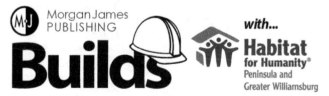

In an effort to support local communities, raise awareness and funds, Morgan James Publishing donates a percentage of all book sales for the life of each book to Habitat for Humanity Peninsula and Greater Williamsburg.

Get involved today! Visit
www.MorganJamesBuilds.com

This book is dedicated to my clients. Without your courage, compassion, and insight, this book wouldn't be possible.

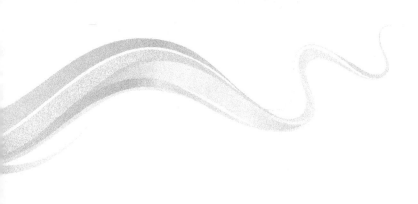

contents

lighter

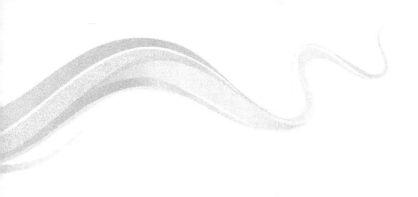

CHAPTER ONE

You Can Begin Feeling Lighter Now

I want you to imagine for a moment that you are at your goal weight, wearing your favorite clothes, laughing and smiling, and doing what it is you most want to be doing with your life.

Yes – you're at your goal weight, but it's so much more than that. Nothing is holding you back. You do what you want and go where you want. Yes, you take the trip to Mexico or Italy and you can walk and spend all day out enjoying yourself. You have sustainable, ongoing energy. You *feel* light and free. Your mind and heart are lighter as well – free from thinking about food or worrying about your weight. There's a lightness in your step, you walk taller, and smoother – more agile. Everything you do is easier. And you're doing the things you love to do since you're not thinking about food nor planning meals all day long.

It's your dream come true, and your first step starts right now.

Keeping that vision in mind, I want you to give yourself some credit for all the hard work you've already done to lose weight. You may think that it's all been futile – because if it weren't, you wouldn't be reading this book right now – but that's not entirely true.

You've learned a lot about how to lose weight, and likely lost a lot of weight in your past, yet it always came back.

Knowing *how to lose weight* but not being able to follow through on that knowing in a consistent way can be very frustrating, and I imagine – since you're reading this book – you know what I'm referring to.

It's knowing that you should eat a healthy dinner, yet on the way home after a busy and stressful day and realizing you don't have anything prepared, you stop by your favorite take-out instead.

It's knowing that if you could just get up that extra 30 minutes earlier, you'd be able to get in that workout, and thinking about your treadmill at home which has become more like a hanger for discarded clothing.

It's looking in the fridge at the apple, and reaching for the cheesecake.

It's making sure everyone else is happy, before you can relax, then realizing it's a never-ending battle pleasing everyone.

It's feeling judged for your physical size, and feeling insecure and inadequate for not being able to do something that seems easy enough to do ahead of time, but impossible in the moment.

It's almost worse – knowing what to do, but regularly doing the opposite.

And all that is about to change for you – so hold on. Just as it changed for my new client, Laura.

Laura arrived at the hypnosis office for her group session. I wasn't surprised to hear her describe feeling frustrated about not following through on what she knows she needs to do to lose weight and keep it off for life.

"I just don't know what to do," she said.

"I eat healthy food! But I can't seem to lose weight and keep it off – and nothing seems to work, so I stop trying. And I know I need to exercise more."

She continued to describe how she's aware of what she *should* be doing – but her mom was ill, and her son was going through a rough time – it's hard for her to actually do those things with any consistency.

And these issues she's describing are real life issues – they're not excuses. Her mom being ill means excess worry about her health, and time out of her day driving her mom to appointments and specialists. Her son going through a rough time means worrying about him and his happiness, and going out of her way to do anything that could help him.

Laura's scenario is common – knowledge and desire to lose weight, but a lack of time, energy, and follow-through to make it happen.

She continued with: "I eat a healthy breakfast and lunch, but by the time I get home from work all I want to do is relax with my husband – so I eat too much, then more after dinner. It doesn't matter what I've planned for the day, by the time I get home, I'm too tired to walk or cook something healthy. And half the time I'm dealing with my mom's caregivers or worrying about my son. It feels like I'm barely hanging in there. And on top of all that, work is very stressful and I get terrible sleep."

Laura has stress upon stress upon stress. She's intelligent, successful, and at least on the surface has a lot of things going for her – a great job, a good family, and financial security.

And yet there's always something deeper going on, something that precipitated this meeting, on this day. Just as you decided to read this book now – so I asked Laura what I always ask my clients – a question that I want you to consider as well:

"Why are you here today?" I asked her. And for you, it's "Why read this book now?"

"Because," she said, "when I look in the mirror I see my mom. And she's struggling so much right now with her health and weight, and I don't want my life to be like that. I'm scared."

"I'm so glad you're here," I told her, "because I know I can help you." While this may sound like only Laura's problem, I see this all the time in my group sessions. Women and men who know *how* to lose weight, but are unable to follow through on their plans in a consistent way to keep the weight off. And the first thing I teach them is that we're trained to eat wrong.

WE'RE TRAINED TO EAT WRONG

It's not your fault I share with my groups – ***you were trained to eat wrong.*** From an early age, many kids are given specific times to eat, and are instructed to eat food that they either don't want, or aren't hungry for. Do any of these sound familiar to you?

Eat a healthy breakfast – it's the most important meal of the day.

Finish everything on your plate – there are starving children in Africa (or China).

You don't get to leave the table until you finish your dinner.

Don't you want to grow up to be healthy and strong? Eat everything on your plate.

Add to that specific times of the day for lunch and dinner, regardless of hunger levels, and over time we are trained out of our natural instinct for food – which is to eat when we feel the sensation of hunger and to stop eating when we're no longer hungry.

Let me ask you something – how do you know when it's time to go to the bathroom?

(Note: This question usually results in looks of confusion and curiosity.)

Do you schedule it, like at 8 am every day, then at noon, you're going to go to the bathroom?

No, *that's right*, you feel it. You know it's time to go to the bathroom when you feel it in your body, and that's the same thing we need to do with eating, but for most of us, we're trained to ignore that signal and we eat according to other factors for most of our lives.

There are good reasons why our parents and teachers want kids to eat at certain times of the day – it would be harder on the adults to raise kids and allow them to eat whenever they wanted – but as we get older, when we're living on our own, when we're adults, we need a better way of eating. We need to listen to our body and eat according to what it's asking for.

WHY DIETS DON'T WORK

The ***problem with diets*** is that they are energy driven – meaning you need to put a certain amount of regular energy into sticking with your diet. There's an overhead cost to counting, weighing, or pointing foods, and for most people, they can stick with it for a while, but once things get stressful, the diet goes out the window, and more pounds come flying in as a result.

The other problem with most diets is that they require what we call "will power" to stay on track. This means there's some level of deprivation – we're hungry, but we don't eat. Does that make sense to you? Would it make sense to not go to the bathroom when you feel it? It's against our natural design, so it doesn't work in the long run.

Would it make sense to feel the sensation for going to the bathroom, and look at the clock or a schedule and realize – no, it's not *time* for me to go to the bathroom yet! I just went to the bathroom an hour ago! I have to wait! That doesn't make sense, and neither does eating when you're not hungry.

The other issue with most diets is that they're not feasible or realistic to be sustainable for the long term. This is why so many people can lose weight while they're on their diet, but the moment they're not on their diet anymore, the weight creeps back – usually with a few extra pounds.

This adds frustration, and feelings of guilt and worthlessness for most people.

The reality is, when we have what I call stored energy on the body, our appetite is suppressed because the body doesn't actually want us to be overweight. It's not economical for the body to carry excess weight around.

When we give our body an opportunity, it will self-regulate, *which means your appetite is suppressed, you eat less, and lose weight.*

And there are ways to facilitate that natural process of consistent weight loss using hypnosis and by knowing the way the body and brain actually work.

You may be thinking this is all well and good but can you really break your habits of eating? Yes, you can, and as we get into the book I'm going to show you how. I've helped hundreds of men and women who were ready to lose weight by ending end the cycle of emotional eating and begin feeling lightness – by both being in control of food and losing weight without the struggle.

Before we get into the details, it's important that you know what your brain actually needs for permanent weight loss.

WHAT OUR BRAIN ACTUALLY NEEDS FOR PERMANENT WEIGHT LOSS

I'm going to tell you what actually works, in my experience – and there's significant research supporting it as well – the field of neuroscience is backing up what I'm going to share with you about what the brain is doing.

In the simplest terms, the brain always turns away from pain and toward pleasure. There are many primary functions of the brain, one is to keep us safe, and another is to optimize the\physical aspects of our body for efficiency and to conserve energy – so the body wants to preserve energy wherever it can, and remain basically in a peaceful state wherever it can. The brain would rather be at peace than excited – it's called homeostasis, and it's the brain's desire to remain in balance.

What this means, is that when you're not feeling well – you're stressed, or bored – your brain doesn't like it. Your brain will **always, without failure, try to bring you back to homeostasis (balance) using any means possible.**

This means, if you don't have any other mechanism in place to bring peace to your heart and mind, your brain will get it elsewhere, and food is a really easy short-term solution to this problem with a very high long-term cost.

So, what your brain actually needs for permanent weight loss is for you to listen to your body – eat only when you're hungry, and have some way of bringing your brain back into peaceful balance when it's stressed. If you have no other way of doing that than with food, well, then you are very likely to gain weight.

Here are the two most important rules for permanent weight loss:

1. Eat only when you're actually hungry.
2. Do things that naturally generate good feelings. Those good feelings are what your brain is looking for when it reaches for the cheesecake instead of the salad, or when you have a desire for donuts instead of heading out on a walk.

It *can* be that simple. Those two things are all the brain wants in order to self-regulate and return to a healthy weight. Not super-model skinny by the way. We talked about stored energy on the body – it's like a savings account of energy for the body, aka fat. Well the body wants some energy in its bank account. This system is not about getting unnaturally thin – it's about a healthy weight for you, a feeling of lightness in your heart, mind, and body.

Together, we'll come up with a system that helps your brain and body realign with what works for you so that you eat only when you're hungry, and so that you're able to bring your body to a peaceful, comfortable state and do that with regularity and consistency. And hypnosis facilitates that process and basically helps us to make this switch infinitely faster than just trying to do it alone.

HOW IT WORKS:

There are three phases to the approach that naturally build upon each other to enable weight loss to become easier over time.

Phase 1: Simple Weight Loss

The first phase of permanent weight loss is learning how to consistently lose weight week after week, and – most importantly – do it in a way that is sustainable for the rest of your life.

Simple means only focusing on a few things, and that those things are easy to understand. And so for phase 1, there is only one thing to do which will be repeated over and over:

Only eat when you are *actually* hungry.

Not for emotional reasons, not for pure pleasure, not because someone else is eating or wants you to. Eat only when you're actually hungry. Actually hungry is the challenge, and implementing that day in and day out is where the work is involved.

Every client in groups I work with has unique strengths and challenges – things they're doing well, and areas they can improve on. This is not a cookie-cutter approach, and that is by design. For anything to help you lose weight and keep it off for life, it must be something you can easily do for the long term.

Phase 2: Easy Weight Loss

When you think of phase 2, I want you to think about optimizing what is working well and fine-tuning it so it's enjoyable and repeatable. Easy weight loss is achievable by incorporating habits and techniques that actually work for you that you also enjoy and provide repeatable results.

The goal of phase 2 is *not* to help you lose weight as quickly as possible, the goal is to help you lose weight *as quickly as makes sense for you given your circumstances*. There will be some aspects and tools in the easy phase that make perfect sense for you because they're relatively easy – or "low hanging fruit." You can implement them without too much overhead.

There may be other aspects of phase 2 that just don't make sense for you, and it would be better to stick with the simple goal of phase one instead: Only eat when you are actually hungry.

Phase 3: Everlasting Weight Loss

The third phase is specific structure and tools for life-long, permanent weight loss. You'll notice the tools in this chapter are more lifestyle tools to help you feel good and enjoy your life, rather than specific details on how to eat, or how to stay active – and there's a very good reason for that.

Over time, the simplicity and ease of weight loss with hypnosis and the tools and techniques that you use will become habitual, so phase 3 isn't about tools to lose weight – it's about tools to ensure the inevitable stressors of life don't get in the way or knock you off track. It's about emotional well-being for life-long happiness.

In all of these three phases, one of the most important aspects is that the changes and tools are integrated into your life. They must work for you.

HOW THIS BOOK IS ORGANIZED

This book is organized in a way to make both aspects of your brain happy:

The conscious mind, which is analytical and procedural in nature, will love the structured 3 phase approach to permanent weight loss, as well as the detailed 31 specific tools.

The subconscious mind, which is more high-level and associative in nature, will love the holistic concepts of a natural and healthy approach, and also the more dynamic, buffet style of tools and techniques that are flexible for every situation and circumstance.

Hypnosis fits into the process at every level, providing an essential feedback and information gathering tool that gives cohesiveness to the structure and technique to enable simple, easy, and everlasting weight loss.

THE 31 TOOLS

After the chapter on each phase, is a chapter on the tools for that phase. The tools are organized into three categories:

Only Eat When You Are Actually Hungry tools

1. Eat: tools to help you know how, when, and what to eat. These get you back into natural and healthy eating habits so you don't have to *think* about what to do anymore, rather you'll feel it – or know it. You'll naturally only eat when you're actually hungry.

Generate Good Feelings in Your Body tools

2. Move: tools to help motivate you to move your body, and build healthy habits around activity – even if you have physical limitations or challenges. You'll learn why neuroscience is proving the importance of brain health, movement, and permanent weight loss – but you'll likely be surprised by how and why it works.

3. Be: These tools are all about how you are *thinking and feeling* and how to get into a good state of mind. They are probably the most important tools because – when it comes right down to it – we *almost always do what we feel like.* So wouldn't it be nice to feel like doing what you know is good for you already?

Self-mastery of mindful eating – and the Eat category – is of primary importance: Once you only eat when you're hungry, you will lose weight regardless of whether or not you're active enough or feel well. So I consider the move more and feel good components as supportive to eating less. That does not mean they're less important; rather, they support the primary activity of eating less, which is the foundation of continual weight loss.

PUTTING IT ALL TOGETHER

At the end is a blueprint for your success and how to implement the tools right away.

The journey continues now, and I'm so happy that you're coming along for the ride. In the next chapter, I'll describe why hypnosis is an important aspect to weight loss.

Let's begin.

Hypnosis Recording Download

Download your supplemental material including hypnosis audio recordings that accompany this book and program at: LighterBook.com.

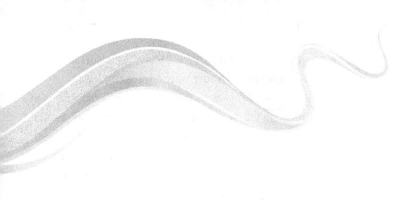

CHAPTER TWO
Why Hypnosis

I wrote this book as a quick reference guide for my clients to use while working with me in my group programs.

I cannot take credit for all of the knowledge and information that I am sharing with you in this book. The ideas regarding how hypnosis works, how the mind works, and how emotions work, came from or were inspired by the work and teachings of Cal Banyan, my teacher. In this book, I add my own insights, tools, and examples to what Cal and other hypnotists teach as well, referenced in the acknowledgment section of this book.

The reality is that most weight loss programs overlook a very important aspect of weight loss – and that's the emotional aspect. So if you've tried things before, and know you're an emotional eater, you've likely been successful to an extent but always fell short in the long run.

My first book, *Reprogram Your Weight*, is a hopeful and thoughtful message full of inspirational client success stories that provide that all-important hope – hope that things can be different.

This book is the roadmap – where you will find the rubber-meets-the-road type of practical application of those ideas outlined in Reprogram Your Weight.

I wrote it as a reference for you to return to regularly, including reviewing the strategy, and the technical components to apply to your life.

Every. Body. Is. Different. Which means the solution for every body – and yes, I'm intentionally spelling it that way – needs a unique solution. This book is a guide toward the unique solution for you that will make sense.

And how do we get to the unique solution for you? With a combination of what you already know with hypnosis to reveal the root issues and transform habits. Hypnosis also amplifies what is working by creating positive feedback loops in the brain that we experience as natural motivation.

I hope that you will read it, then refer back to it to check in and adjust as you improve in your ability to make the changes you want to make, but also when anything stressful or unexpected comes up in life. There's a technique applicable for nearly every situation.

I wrote it to help you know that even if you have tried everything else – hypnosis still works.

And you may be wondering, "But what exactly is hypnosis, and how and why does it work?"

WHY HYPNOSIS

One of the most important things about hypnosis that I want you to be aware of is that it is a normal and natural state of mind.

You've likely been in a state of hypnosis thousands of times in your life. It's as natural as being happy, or intrigued.

Hypnosis is a state of heightened and focused awareness. In this state, you become aware of things that you weren't aware of before, which leads to important insights about your life and the ability to more easily make changes you want to make.

Other terms that are associated with hypnosis include an athlete being "in the zone," or when someone is "in flow," or even just pure presence. They are all states of altered consciousness that can provide us with tremendous value.

The common thread between all of those states of mind is the ability to be in that moment – even if in that moment you are highly focused on something you want to happen in the future, or are healing from something in the past.

But why and how does that actually happen? To answer that question, it will help to think of the mind as having different aspects, or parts. The two parts that are important to understand are: the conscious mind, and the subconscious mind.

THE CONSCIOUS MIND

The conscious mind, referred to from here on out as CM, is analytical and procedural. It's the part of your mind that thinks linearly. It's our point of focus – whatever you are focused on right now is what the conscious mind is doing.

So as you read or listen to this book, you are consciously focusing on it using the conscious mind. If you're spacing off while trying to read, your conscious mind is off daydreaming or thinking about something else.

But the conscious mind is very limited. Studies indicate the conscious mind can only hold onto about seven pieces of information at any one time. This means the conscious mind, although powerful, important, and beneficial, is limited in its capacity to solve big problems.

WHY YOU SHOULD CARE

I know you're probably thinking, *why does this matter – I just want to lose weight!* And here's why – if what you're focused on is something that does not feel good – meaning you're feeling sad, bored, or lonely for example, your conscious mind will purposefully try to get you to focus on doing something else to feel better. And if the only thing you know how to do to feel better is eat, and if you have unresolved emotional turmoil in your life, then your conscious mind will regularly be giving you the idea to eat food, to distract yourself from those bad feelings in an attempt to feel better.

THE SUBCONSCIOUS MIND

The subconscious mind (SCM) is vast and unlimited in capacity. Instead of being linear and analytical like the CM, the SCM is associative, and expansive. It is where all of our feelings and emotions reside, and it retains a memory of everything that ever happened to us.

The conscious mind helps us to focus, and the subconscious mind helps us to expand, find associations, and makes connections with things that we didn't realize were related.

So anytime we're unable to solve an issue in our life by focusing on it, it's usually a good indicator that the subconscious mind is an effective tool for the job.

WE ALMOST ALWAYS DO WHAT WE *FEEL* LIKE

Have you ever wondered, how is it that you can *know* (conscious mind) what to do, yet not follow through consistently?

The reason is that we almost always do what we *feel* (subconscious mind) like. And when we do something but don't want to – we'll often complain about it and say things like "Fine, I'll do it but I don't feel like it!"

This concept cannot be stressed enough, because – guess what – if you always felt like eating healthy and exercising, you probably wouldn't be having this issue.

The subconscious mind is where that feeling comes from. So if you know what you want to do, but don't feel like doing it, then there's a disconnect, an incongruence. And within that incongruence lies the answer to why you can know what you want to do, yet not follow through.

WHY IT MATTERS

Hypnosis unlocks the door to that solution. Hypnosis is what gives us direct access to the SCM and provides the reasons for why we don't feel like doing things, gives us the ability to resolve those issues, then reprogram a new way of thinking and being that we actually want.

A Leaky Roof Issue

I like to use the analogy of a leaky roof to describe how hypnosis works.

I think everyone can agree that a leaky roof is not a good thing, I suppose unless you're a roofer. Setting that aside, a leaky roof is not a good thing. It can be expensive, time-consuming, and stressful - yet it's also important to note that you really can't successfully ignore a leaky roof either. It will tend to get worse over time, and cause more problems.

Think of your weight loss as the leaky roof.

Now imagine that you go up into your attic with a flashlight to take a look at your roof to find the leak. The flashlight is your conscious mind. It's focused, but limited. You see water on the inside of your roof, and so, using the tools that you find in the bookstore, online, and from friends, you patch up that leak.

And it's dry for a few weeks.

Until it rains really hard again a month later (aka stress), and it's leaking again.

This time you get up on your roof, and again, address the issue by taking a close look at where it appears the leak is coming through. Again you are focused, and you patch up that area of the roof – this time from the outside, and the leak stops and dries up.

Until a few weeks later, when again it rains really hard and your roof is leaking.

By this point you're getting really frustrated because you've worked on your roof from the inside, you've worked on it from the outside. You asked all your friends, and you understand how gravity works, and you didn't see anything else that needed to be fixed. But it's still leaking.

So, you talk to a roofer who resolves these types of issues all the time.

When the roofer comes to your home, they don't just bring a flashlight into the attic, they bring a flood light, and light the entire room. They not only look at the leaky, wet spot on top of your roof, but they check the gutters, and all the other parts of your roof as well.

They look at the roof from a holistic point of view – which is what the SCM does. Once the floodlight is turned on, you see there are a few other wet spots pouring into the primary leak that you didn't notice with your flashlight. Upon further investigation, your roofer notices that the primary drain on your roof was plugged up, and water was leaking under a part of your roof! After the drain was cleared, the roof didn't leak again, because it was draining properly as it should have.

The subconscious mind does the same thing for us – provides us more information in an expansive and holistic way that helps to describe where we may have issues keeping us from being successful.

HYPNOSIS REVEALS THE ISSUE, THEN FACILITATES INSIGHT AND TRANSFORMATION

One of the fascinating things about hypnosis is the following: Hypnosis is not the key to solving your problems. Rather, hypnosis is a tool that helps to *reveal then facilitate resolving the issue.*

This is important, because the point is that hypnosis is not magic. It's a normal and natural state of mind that we go into all the time. And working with a hypnosis professional – all it means, is that they can help bring you into that normal and natural state of mind *on purpose to get expected and repeatable results.*

The process of hypnosis – including making associations, and gaining an expanded view – give you more information and insight into your issue.

More information than you had before. Just like with the leaky roof. If you knew it was your clogged gutter, you'd just go unclog it. And you've likely tried everything you can think of – but it's still not enough. That's a sign that the answer for you is bigger than what your conscious mind can do. Basically, your conscious mind isn't the tool for the job.

And with hypnosis, we can do the same thing with whatever it is that is keeping you from being able to do what makes sense for you to lose weight and keep it off for the rest of your life.

Sometimes the issue is a painful experience in your life, whether you're consciously aware of it or not. Abandonment, abuse, neglect, or feeling unloved or unwanted. And guess what – your brain does not like those painful feelings, and it will do anything at all to keep you from experiencing them. Even if it means distracting you with food to the point that the excess weight becomes its own painful issue.

And that is where hypnosis really shines, because not only can it identify the issue, but in that highly resourceful and expansive state of association, it facilitates the transformation of painful feelings and memories into more useful feelings. Think of an old scar on your hand; most people have cut themselves at least once while cooking. Look at that scar. You know it hurt. But it also healed, and maybe you learned something in the process, maybe not, but it healed – you know it happened, but it's not ruining your life. Hypnosis doesn't erase painful memories; it sets you free from them by transforming them into something better and you end up feeling emotionally lighter in the process. And guess what happens when you experience emotional lightness? Your physical body wants to catch up.

So what does the process actually look like? In the next chapter we dive into the details of Phase 1: Simple Weight Loss.

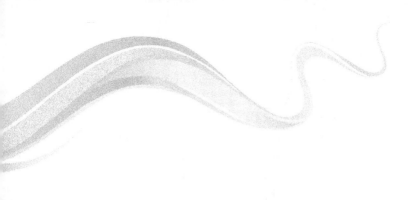

CHAPTER THREE
Phase 1: Simple Weight Loss

The key to everlasting weight loss is to simplify it as much as possible by coming up with a plan that seamlessly fits into your life – with all of the current struggles and stress, in a way that is sustainable over the long term.

Not a plan that expects your life to become less stressful, or easier. Not a plan that requires hours at the gym, or a complicated food plan.

And for that reason, it's important to have a unique plan for every client. There are foundational aspects that in general, work for everyone, then there are custom tools that each client will find works best for them, given their current situation.

This means that for someone who's retired, they'll find certain tools useful, and another client, stressed out with work and life, will find different tools useful.

This chapter describes the foundation of consistent weight

loss applicable to nearly everyone, then the next chapter includes the tools to implement for your unique situation.

Put Away the Scale

The scale is a source of so many bad feelings. Depending on what it says on any particular day, it can make us feel great, or terrible. The scale itself is a poor instrument for measuring our overall health, and it also does a poor job of telling us how we're doing with regards to our weight loss goals. In my experience, it tends to make people feel bad, not good.

In my group workshops, it comes up a lot that people are reluctant to put away their scale – how would they know how they were doing, they ask?

So I ask them if the scale, and weighing themselves is actually working – does it lead to the weight loss they are looking for? No, they reply.

For now, don't weigh yourself. You'll know how well you're doing based on your behavior – the ability to eat only when you're actually hungry, and feel good about it. You'll likely stop thinking about food so much within the first week, and feel more relaxed and happy.

Applying the Two Most Important Things for Permanent Weight Loss

Remember the two most important things from chapter 1?

1. *Eat only when you are actually hungry.*

2. *Generate good feelings in your body.*

This is where we learn how to actually do those things.

1. Only Eat When You're Actually Hungry, aka Mindful Eating

The body knows how to regulate your weight and appetite, but since we're trained out of listening to our body to know when it's time to eat, we end up eating at the wrong times, and end up eating for reasons other than actual hunger. Fixing this one problem helps people lose weight and keep it off for life. The challenge is in the implementation.

Why do we eat?

Habit: eating in front of the television, or eating at 9 am every day.

Societal pressure: eating because the food is in the break room, or you were invited to a party.

Now or never: eating because if you don't now, you won't be able to later.

Emotional reasons: eating because you're feeling bored, sad, lonely, depressed.

Pleasure: eating because it tastes good and is pleasurable.

Hunger: eating because you're actually hungry, and your body is asking for food.

What I've discovered in working with hundreds of clients is that in general, most are just eating way too much food.

At the end of my group sessions, I'll ask clients 3 questions:

How easy was this for you?

They always reply something like, easier than I thought possible. Some clients actually think there's something wrong, that it has to be hard to lose weight, but that's not true.

Do you think you could do this for the rest of your life?

The answer is always, "Yes."

How much food are you eating now, in comparison to before we began working together?

The answer is between 25-50% of the amount of food they used to eat! Isn't that incredible? We're just eating way too much food. This comes from large portions at restaurants which skew our perception of a normal serving of food.

A note on the term "mindful eating": Mindful eating may be different than what you're thinking, so if you've heard this term before, know that this is a custom concept for the work I do with clients and in my groups.

Mindful eating is a very simple concept that can take months to master. Here it is:

Only Eat When You Are Actually Hungry.

This means you don't eat according to the clock, or a set schedule, or because breakfast is the most important meal of the day.

That style of eating is using our conscious mind to understand when it's time to eat, rather than allowing our physical body to signal that it's time to eat.

Here's how I explain it to workshop participants:

The four most important things:

1. Have healthy food available to you at all times – at home, the office, and while traveling.

2. Then, wait for the signal from your body – it will be a feeling in your stomach area like a growling stomach, or a ping type feeling in your stomach area. Note that this can take getting used to if you've been ignoring it most of your life.

3. Once you have the signal from your stomach, eat within 30 minutes.

4. Take about 1/2 the amount of food that you're accustomed to having – you can always go back for more.

More detail:

- If you wait too long to eat, your blood sugar will drop which kicks off a fear-based response in your body and you will always overeat.

- I'll repeat that: Eat within 30 minutes because if you wait you will always overeat.

- With every bite of food, you're asking yourself – am I still hungry? One way to think about this, is "If I weren't sitting here already eating, would I think I'm hungry?"

- Stop when you're no longer hungry. Even if it means you're in mid-bite.

- Put the food back, or throw it away. Keep in mind that if you keep eating when you're not hungry, your body will process it and it will be stored as fat by your liver. This means, if you feel "bad" about wasting food, then how you really need to fix it is to take less.

- You're either throwing your food away into a

regular garbage can, where it can be consumed by little bugs and gets put back into the earth, or you're throwing it into the garbage can of your body. The best way to resolve this issue is to take less.

- You'll be surprised how much less you need, but keep in mind that you have stored energy on your body.
- Always serve your own food so you can take the right portion.
- You may have heard something like if you don't eat every few hours, your metabolism will slow. This is not true. If you put food in your body when it's not asking for food – it gets stored as fat. What do you think knows what's better for your body – a book, or your own stomach and brain?
- Mindful eating is like a bull's eye, and in the first week, I just want you to hit the wall that the bull's eye is attached to. Over time it will become automatic, and you won't need to think about it so much anymore.
- You will naturally eat only when hungry over time, and this becomes your new normal.
- Imagine you're at an event, and someone walks by with a tray of your favorite food – when you're eating mindfully, you won't even notice the food go by, because you're not hungry.
- Are you the only one putting food into your

mouth? If so, then you have complete control over this, and keep in mind, this is the conscious expectation and plan for you. If this were easy to do, you'd do it all on your own but what is usually happening is that there's a high level of emotional eating (eating because of stress, boredom, or any other feeling that isn't hunger), and bad habits.

- This retrains your brain to eat only when hungry. And when that happens, you'll be eating less food, and begin losing weight consistently.

- Keep in mind that too much healthy food is still too much food. You can gain weight by eating too many salads.

A NOTE ON SUGAR

Sugar is processed differently in the body. It's like a drug, so eating lots of carbs and sugar will not give us a full feeling, and when eating too many carbs and sugar, you can get the insulin response which leads to cravings and feeling like you need to eat every few hours. For that reason, it's important to ensure you're eating more fat than carbs. I recommend replacing sugar and carbs with healthy fats.

WHY IT WORKS:

Automated processes in our body are beating our hearts, regulating our body temperature and blood pressure, and doing all sorts of amazing things on our behalf without us having to do a thing.

Why should we interfere with any of these automated processes? Does a book know more about when you should eat, more than your own body? I don't think so. This is one area where we should be giving the responsibility of knowing when to eat back to our body.

Now sometimes, when we're planning on being in the car for hours or on a plane, we'll go to the bathroom even if we don't feel like we need to go and the same is true for eating. Sometimes you'll need to eat when you're not hungry. But it should still be mindful – meaning it should be something you are choosing on purpose for a specific reason.

You may also choose to eat mindfully and yet still eat a bit of your grandson's birthday cake – but as you'll see in the tools section, a strategy is good to put in place for that – like the two bite strategy.

The job of your conscious mind shifts. Instead of trying to plan when to eat, it now has the job of making sure you always have healthy food available. Then it passes the baton to the body – it will tell you when it's time to eat.

Don't worry if you don't know what hunger feels like; it will come back to you and you'll get better at it over time – just like anything we do – with practice, we get better.

If you're on a certain medication that impacts your appetite, adjustments can be made.

The next step in phase one is to begin generating good feelings in the body so that you won't need to reach for that donut or ice cream to feel good.

2. GENERATE GOOD FEELINGS IN YOUR BODY AND MIND

Generating good feelings is doing things that naturally generate the good feeling neurochemicals that our brain needs including: dopamine, serotonin, norepinephrine, endorphins, anandamide, and oxytocin.

When you are naturally generating these feel-good chemicals, your brain is much less likely to reach for sugar or junk food.

When you do not have enough of these feel-good chemicals in your body, your brain will give you ideas about things that will manufacture it – alcohol, smoking, gambling, and of course – food!

This is why, if the only thing you do to feel good is eat, or turn to food to solve every problem, you will likely always have a weight problem and feel out of control to food. This is where the work is involved – finding something else to do other than eat, to make you happy. Now I used the word work because it can take some effort to find and implement these changes but what you're really doing is leading a more happy and fulfilling life in the process, so it's well worth the work to find the things in your life that meet this need.

GENERATE GOOD FEELINGS WITH ACTIVITY

Activity is an important aspect of weight loss – but the rule of thumb when it comes to weight loss is the following: 80% of weight loss is food, and 20% is activity.

You do not have to be active to lose weight. What activity does for us is very important for optimal weight loss and well-being, so I don't want to de-emphasize its role – rather I want you to understand that the most important aspect of weight loss really is eating less, and eating healthier.

- Activity displaces other unhealthy habits like watching TV
- Activity makes us feel good – including dopamine and endorphins

The 1-Minute Rule:

We don't have to have a lot of activity in the day to get the benefits from it. And the 1-minute rule makes it easy for our brains to handle – we don't get stressed out thinking about doing it for one minute. If you don't have one minute a day to be active, even just 30 seconds out the door, and 30 seconds back, then you have a different problem – meaning you're too busy, and that needs to be addressed first.

GENERATE GOOD FEELINGS BY LEARNING TO RELAX

Our body needs relaxation which is really about rejuvenation – recharging the body. Most clients are too stressed, and there's an undercurrent of anxiety in everything they do.

Why it works:

Learning to relax, only 12 minutes a day, can provide the body with the recharge it needs to be fully optimized throughout the day. And this is like practice: the more you learn to relax with hypnosis, the easier it is for your body to recharge in any situation. For me personally, I know all I need is about 10 minutes in the day of self-hypnosis to bring myself back up to feeling 100%.

- Download your *Learning to Relax* Hypnosis audio recording that accompanies this book at:
- LighterBook.com

GENERATE GOOD FEELINGS WITH DAILY ENJOYMENT

It's so important to have something to look forward to every day. Yet so many of my clients are so busy – and don't feel well in general about themselves – that when they wake up in the morning, they have nothing to look forward to.

This can be as simple as listening to music that you like, or reading. It can be looking at beautiful artwork, or sitting outside and watching the rain fall. It's anything at all that you can honestly say you enjoy. That brings you joy.

Why it works:

For many people in my workshops, the only time they feel good during the day is when they're eating. Period. So of course they're going to overeat! The brain needs to feel good – it's what it wants. *If* you don't give your brain the feel-good feelings, it will find another way to get them, even if it means in the long run you eat too much and gain weight.

GENERATE GOOD FEELINGS WITH HEALTHY SLEEP & DRINKING ENOUGH WATER

Healthy sleep and water are important aspects of consistent weight loss. This does not come as a surprise to most of my clients, and many of them are very good at both of these already. Others need some help.

Why it works:

In order for your body to run optimally, it needs enough sleep and water.

If you're tired, or not sleeping well, it will be harder for you to be successful. This is a no-brainer, and you're probably thinking *duh of course* but I want you to realize two important things:

1. If you're not sleeping well, it will be harder for you to lose weight.
2. The root cause of not sleeping well is very likely the same or related to the issue of weight gain. So they're often addressed and alleviated at the same time with hypnosis.

Bottom line, it's worth paying attention and noticing what can help you sleep better, and if you've already done that, then feel better knowing you'll likely figure it out as part of the process.

If you're dehydrated, what happens is your body basically can't function as well, so it really does slow down your metabolism. What does that really mean? Think of your metabolism as your energy level. It's how energy is processed and distributed in your body. If you don't have enough water – think of it as a backup on the freeway – then your body can't function. It's as if your body turns the dimmer switch on your metabolism. The experience is that you feel tired. And weight loss is stagnant. This is low-hanging fruit, and by that I mean that ensuring you're getting enough water is an easy switch.

How much is enough water? It's different for every person, but if you ever feel tired, or your lips are dry, you waited too long.

The best approach is to drink a pint of water in between meals. Studies indicate that drinking too much with a meal can dilute stomach acids and disrupt digestion. This means you sip water at mealtime, and drink it otherwise.

HOW HYPNOSIS HELPS

Hypnosis helps by relieving any underlying emotional issues causing you to eat when you're not hungry, and also helping to easily switch unhealthy to healthy habits.

PUTTING IT ALL TOGETHER

That's the foundation for consistent weight loss; the next chapter includes specific techniques you can employ to help make the process easy for you.

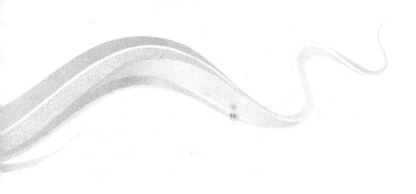

CHAPTER FOUR:

Phase 1: Simple Weight Loss Tools

The tools are organized into 3 categories, based on the foundation of everlasting weight loss:

Only Eat When You're Actually Hungry →
1. Eat Less tools
   Generate Good Feelings →
2. Move More tools
3. Feel Good Tools

EAT LESS TOOLS

1. EAT ONLY WHEN YOU'RE ACTUALLY HUNGRY

This one tool is the foundation for simple and consistent weight loss, but it takes time to rewire the brain to switch from a planned (conscious mind) style eating, to a mindful approach based on when you're actually hungry.

In my first book, Reprogram Your Weight, I recommended the following meme, or hypnotic suggestion:

I eat when I'm hungry, stop when I'm full. Healthy food, in healthy portions.

And I've since updated to the following, based on what I know works better for my clients and group participants. Part of what I do is continually improve my work, which is also outlined in the tool Incremental Success later in this chapter.

I eat only when I'm actually hungry.

I stop when I'm not hungry anymore.

That's it. For every bite of food you put in your mouth, you ask yourself – am I *still* hungry? If not, put the food away and be proud of yourself that you had the awareness to stop when you weren't hungry anymore.

Over time, it will become an automated response – a healthy habit – and you won't need to think about it anymore.

Why the technique changed:

Many clients reported that stopping when full was difficult. And the sensation of "full" for many was actually "stuffed." Scientifically, it takes roughly 20 minutes for us to recognize a sensation of fullness, but for most of my clients it's unrealistic to ask them to slow down, or wait 20 minutes. A better approach is to not wait for the sensation of fullness, rather *notice when the hunger is gone*. It's an approach from a different angle that can be learned, and once in place is extremely valuable. One question to ask yourself is, "If someone asked me right now, 'Are you hungry?' what would you say?" Realize that you may just be eating because the food is in front of you – but you have the control and power to go about it a completely different way.

How hypnosis fits in:

For some people, this is more challenging to do – especially because of emotional eating, so hypnosis helps to eliminate emotional eating, and can also help increase awareness at the trigger point of eating that will help you to easily switch the behavior.

Why it works:

Our bodies are complex and magnificent. Our body knows when it needs food, much more than any book or program can teach us. This is about passing the responsibility of knowing when to eat back to the natural process of our body. This is how we are designed. It works because it's biological and inherent.

Keep in mind that when you're not eating, your body is drawing from stored resources – you're not starving yourself or messing up your metabolism. Your body is burning stored fat – we call it weight loss. You do not need to eat consistently all day long to keep your metabolism up. Rather, you need to eat when your body requests food, aka when you feel hungry.

2. EAT 1/2 SIZE PORTIONS: YOU CAN ALWAYS GO BACK FOR MORE

Start by taking 1/2 size portions. If you're still hungry at the end, then have *half* of the other half.

If your mind or eyeballs hate this idea – or you feel a fear-based anxiety or uncomfortable feeling when you dish up 1/2 size portions, tell yourself, "I can always go back for more." Because in most cases it's true.

How hypnosis fits in:
If this is a challenge and there really is a sense of fear that goes with this, even when knowing you can always go back for more, there may be an underlying emotional trigger that needs to be addressed and resolved.

Why it works:
This technique works because it helps to zero in on the right size portion for you – resetting your default portion size. Over time, you'll notice that you're just eating a lot less – naturally, and it will feel natural to you. You'll feel lighter after you eat, without the heaviness of overeating.

This is a technique that once installed, then becomes the new normal for you, so you won't always take 1/2 size portions – meaning you do not continue to reduce your portions by half. This tool is used at the beginning to reset you to a new portion size that is right for you.

3. AM I HUNGRY? THE BROCCOLI TEST

This technique is designed to help you figure out **if** you're actually hungry. It's useful when you're getting accustomed to mindful eating, but still beneficial for later on when you've got mindful eating down.

Here's how it works:
1.   Think of a food you would **only eat if you're hungry.**
That's why I call it the broccoli test, because for me, I love broccoli but I'll only eat it when I'm hungry. So if I'm standing in front of the fridge looking for something to eat, and I'm not sure if I'm actually hungry or not, I'll ask myself, "Would I eat broccoli?" If the answer is yes, then I'm actually hungry and I'll eat something. If the answer is no, and the only thing that looks or sounds good is ice cream or cookies, I know I'm not actually hungry and that I'm emotionally eating.

1.   If I would eat broccoli, then I'll eat something healthy and follow the rest of the plan.
2.   If I'm not hungry, what it tells me is that my brain wants to feel better. It needs a break from what I'm doing or thinking. This is a signal to do something else. Be grateful that you're noticing this, and don't ignore your body's desire for a break. If you just go back to what you were doing moments earlier (working, worrying, etc.), you'll be back in the kitchen again looking for something.

It's important to remember that when your brain needs something, it will get it one way or the other. If your brain needs a break, it will get one with food, or it will make you feel tired, or you'll begin procrastinating.

Instead, just recognize it for what it is. You have a human body that needs regular breaks and refueling. If you're not hungry, do something else. Listen to music, take a 1-minute walk, or do something else. But it must be enjoyable. Taking a break to fold laundry or do the dishes doesn't work unless you actually get pleasure out of that.

How hypnosis helps:

If it's difficult for you to find something else to do, hypnosis can help with this, and it can also help set a trigger point, or anchor at certain consistent aspects of this issue – for example, even if you put the phrase "Would I eat broccoli?" on your fridge, that could be helpful, but if that's not enough, hypnosis can be used to help figure out where this technique is breaking down and fix it.

Why it works:

This technique works because it gives your brain a meter – a way to test your hunger. It can be very rewarding for the conscious mind to have a tool to understand whether you're actually hungry or not. Having this gauge makes it easy for our brain to know we're doing the right thing, and that makes us feel confident that we're doing the right thing.

4. TRADE CARBOHYDRATES FOR HEALTHY FATS

Studies continue to prove that carbohydrates do not contribute to healthy weight loss, rather we should be eating more healthy fat. But how does that actually work?

One of the best ways is to reduce the carbohydrates in your diet with fat. For example, if you have a bagel with peanut butter in the morning, you'd switch that to half to begin with (1/2 size portions technique), then have more peanut butter and less bagel.

How hypnosis helps:

A common myth, perpetuated by bad science and a scandal, indicated for decades that saturated fat caused heart disease. This means that for many of us, we grew up in an environment where fat was the enemy, and believing that fat made us fat. But it's not true – in fact, all the latest research indicates it's sugar that makes us fat. Yet a lifelong belief that fat is the enemy can be hard to just switch consciously. Hypnosis can help update this limiting belief so that you don't feel bad about eating healthy fat.

Why it works:

There's tremendous research indicating why fat is better for our bodies than carbohydrates, but I like to use the following analogy instead:

Imagine a campfire. The campfire represents your metabolism, and the flames and fire represent available energy to you in the body.

Processed carbohydrates and sugar are like putting tissue paper on the fire – a quick flare up, then it dissipates. You'll feel hungry again quickly. You're left with a mess of ash (unhealthy residue) in the body. This is the same as what sugar does to our body – raises our blood sugar, then it crashes.

Complex / natural carbs, including things like fruit and vegetables, are like kindling. Useful for immediate energy, and lasts longer. Less residue.

Fat is like a presto log. It burns slowly, continually for a long time. You don't feel the need to eat again for a while, and there's minimal residue.

5. HAVE HEALTHY FOOD AVAILABLE AT ALL TIMES

Planning is an important aspect of simple and consistent weight loss because if you don't have food available to you when you're hungry, you will very likely overeat when you do have food available, or eat the wrong foods.

This is how it works:
Have healthy food available at all times. This means at home, at work, in the car, while traveling, everywhere.

This means you'll need to spend at least an hour every week going to the grocery store making sure you have this healthy food available for you at all times.

There is an overhead cost to the planning and prepara-tion. But this overhead cost is minimal in comparison to what it will get for you. Plus, the conscious mind really wants to be involved in the process of continual weight loss and planning and list creation is a conscious mind activity.

A few of the foods that I end up recommending to my clients over and over include raw, unsalted nuts – including almonds – and small bits of cheese.

How hypnosis helps:
Hypnosis helps by giving this job to the conscious mind. The conscious mind, being analytical and procedural, wants to be involved in the process of weight loss. The conscious mind loves the planning aspect and so, if it is hard for you to find time to do the planning, hypnosis can help prioritize this aspect; without it, you'll find yourself eating the wrong foods at the wrong times because you haven't done proper planning.

Why it works:
Planning is an important part of most things that we are successful at. We plan a lot of things in life – to go to school, to finish a project, to save money. We plan vacations. And we need to plan out our food as well. Because with our busy lives, by the time we get hungry – knowing that you overeat if you don't eat within 30 minutes – it means if you don't have healthy food with you, you're very likely to eat the wrong foods or overeat.

6: HOW WILL I FEEL IN 2 HOURS?

This tool is all about truth in advertising. I discussed this in my first book, *Reprogram Your Weight*.

Imagine that advertisers were required to put on the front of products how you were likely to feel 2 hours after you eat it.

What would the bag of chips look like – you with low energy and sluggish.

How about that carton of ice cream – feeling guilty and tired?

Here's how the tool works, and to begin with, only do this if you have a problem food that you want to get out of your life. It's not necessary for all foods, because once you start eating healthier, you will naturally gravitate toward the healthier foods.

Step 1: Write down the problem food. Be specific. If it's a bag of chips, write down the name of the chips, and the size.

Step 2: Imagine yourself 2 hours after consuming the chips. What are you doing? Are you sitting in front of the television? Are you on your computer? Imagine taking a selfie 2 hours after eating that food, and what comes with it.

Step 3: Write down what the cover of that food should look like. For example, if it were a bag of chips, imagine the bag of chips says "Feel Guilty!" on the front, with a picture of you falling asleep in front of the TV.

How hypnosis helps:

Hypnosis can help associate you into how you actually feel after consuming problem foods. It facilitates and empowers this process.

Why it works:

For problem foods, what happens is the brain is associating only the initial sensation of the food – how delicious it is, and the beneficial chemicals released when you eat that delicious food – with that food. It has neglected to connect the dots to that end point – how it actually makes you feel in the long run.

So by incorporating the truth about how that food actually makes you feel, you are more easily able to avoid that food in your future – it's simply not as attractive to you anymore.

This technique works really well for problem foods, but is not recommended for large groups of food. In my experience, it works well for specific types of ice cream, specific types of chips, and specific types of cookies or crackers. And the brain does a great job of generalizing, so once you do this for one food and it's no longer attractive to you anymore, your brain will find other associations with other foods that make sense to apply this same technique to.

MOVE MORE TOOLS

7. ONE MINUTE OF ACTIVITY PER DAY

This is a very useful tool that I recommend to all of my clients, although if they are already accustomed to exercise, I may increase the duration.

Here's how it works:

I want you to get some type of activity in every single day. That's right. Every single day… for one minute.

One minute of walking, or some other type of activity. It can be as simple as walking out your door for 30 seconds, and turning around and coming back inside.

After a week, double it to 2 minutes.

After another week double it again.

Pretty soon you'll be up to 10 minutes per day of activity which feels really good for your heart, brain, and body.

If you're already doing some type of regular activity, drop the duration and increase the consistency. This needs to be Every. Single. Day. That's what's important, and it's also why 1-minute works so well for people: Because you can always do more and in many cases the hardest part of being active is getting started. We often talk ourselves out of the 30 minutes on the treadmill, but 30 seconds out the door and back is much easier. And at times, once you're out the door, you'll go longer. So the one minute can turn into 5 without any big issue.

How hypnosis helps:

Hypnosis can help create a healthy habit here, and also help to determine what type of activity can make the most sense for consistent application. The key here is consistency, and that's why if nothing else, just walk for one minute.

Why it works:

Consistency is the trick as to why 1-minute works so well for people, because you can always do more and in many cases, the hardest part of being active is getting started.

Over time you'll realize you've created a very healthy habit of getting in some activity – even if it's just a minute, even on your busiest days. This leads to you being more active in other areas of your life – yet it feels natural, not forced.

FEEL GOOD TOOLS

8. HAVE FUN AND ENJOYMENT DAILY

The brain wants to feel good. If it doesn't feel good, or needs a break, it will give you the idea for anything at all that does feel good, and for many people wanting to lose weight, the thing that does feel good is eating. And for many people that is *the only thing that feels good, so the brain has no other choice.*

How it works:
Find something else to do that you enjoy, as many things as possible, and incorporate them into your life.

Some should be really easy – a no-brainer. They should require as much effort as eating ice cream. This is important, because if your only enjoyment is golfing or sailing, you won't feel like doing that when you're tired, and you'll find yourself back in front of the fridge eating again.

Here are a few common things that people do, but you'll need to find your own:

- Listen to music
- Play an instrument
- Read
- Watch a favorite TV show (no food allowed)
- Listen to a podcast
- Go for a walk
- Sew, knit, needlepoint
- Do something artistic: photography, painting, pottery
- Gardening
- Go for a drive or ride
- Working in the shop – wood, cars, building something
- Puzzles: a real, classic puzzle on the kitchen table, or a crossword puzzle or sudoku
- Playing a game on your phone
- Writing, but only if you enjoy it
- Those are just a few ideas. Write down what works for you, and fill your home with things you enjoy.

How hypnosis helps:

Hypnosis can help you to intentionally create more joy in your life by helping you to find things you enjoy doing, and anchoring in these elements when necessary.

Why it works:

Plan on doing something enjoyable every single day. Over time, you'll have more than just food that brings you peace or enjoyment. Pretty soon your brain has multiple options for taking a break or getting some feel-good brain chemicals, and now you're no longer in the kitchen looking for food. Instead you're doing things you love.

9. RELAX DAILY, INCLUDING WITH HYPNOSIS

Just as the mind needs enjoyment daily, it also needs a way to consistently relax and recharge with or without hypnosis.

There are two ways that work for this:

1. Do No Thing

Do No Thing is about giving yourself the freedom and permission to just sit there and not intentionally do anything at all. The key to this technique is to realize that while you are doing No Thing, your body is doing all sorts of automated things on your behalf. You're effectively giving your body an opportunity to recharge. So think of it as you are plugging in your battery, and recharging.

How to do it:

Sit down, hopefully in a quiet space, and do No Thing for 5 minutes. No email, no TV, no work, no reading. No intentional thinking, or anything at all. Self-hypnosis or light music are fine, so tools 9 and 10 are often combined.

2. Self-Hypnosis

The other way to relax daily includes self-hypnosis. Instead of Do No Thing, you purposefully do self-hypnosis.

Hypnosis is a tool that you can use for a variety of

purposes, and self-hypnosis is the ability for you to learn to use hypnosis on your own to gain important insights about yourself, and basically optimize every area of your life.

One of the easiest ways to do self-hypnosis is to get in a comfortable position where you will remain undisturbed for 12 minutes. Set the timer on your phone or other device so you're not tempted to look at what time it is.

Next, close your eyes and take in a nice deep breath all the way to your toes. Imagine a color that represents feeling relaxed and tranquil. Imagine breathing that color to the tips of your toes.

Now imagine a color that represents stress, anxiety, and everything you no longer need, like toxins.

Imagine exhaling out that color.

Now putting it all together, you breathe in the color of relaxation to your toes, and exhale out the color of everything you no longer need.

Moving up your body now, you relax your feet and exhale out.

Next, you relax your legs.

Do this all the way up your body.

Why it works:

Because the breathing, color, and going up your body helps to focus your mind which helps you relax. Now to be clearer, hypnosis is not relaxation. But this particular hypnosis is about relaxation. In the hypnosis office, there are all sorts of different types of hypnosis techniques we'll use to get you the desired results.

How hypnosis helps:

Do No Thing can be hard for some people, especially if they have a lot of thoughts, or are very stressed. Hypnosis can alleviate that stress and out-of-control thinking to enable Do No Thing in a way that is very comfortable.

Why it works:

The body needs to recharge. And when we recharge we feel better. So much of our day is filled with stress and tension, and the opposite of that is relaxation. This does not mean you're going to the spa or getting a massage, it means you're getting out of your own way. Do No Thing, and allow the body to rebalance itself – take itself back into homeostasis.

10. N-STATE

N-State is a play on words created by accident. I was sharing the following with a colleague, and she thought I said "N-State," and it stuck. It represents the following two concepts:

End-State: The state of mind you'll be in when you accomplish your weight loss goals and everything related to it.

In-State: Being in the state of mind *now* of your end-state.

How to do it:

Step 1: Benefits of the change

Write down at least 5 benefits of weight loss on a piece of paper. Some will likely include things like feeling lighter, feeling more in control, fitting in my clothes, but they should also include other elements related to health and how you feel. For example: Reduce or eliminate medication, sleep better, have more energy.

Step 2: Self Hypnosis

Get in a comfortable position where you can remain undisturbed for at least 10 minutes.

Note: Download your N-State Hypnosis Worksheet and accompanying hypnosis audio recording at : LighterBook.com.

Begin with the basic self-hypnosis technique.

Step 3: End-State

Imagine that you are at some point in your future. You're at your goal weight, but it's more than that.

You have more energy, and feel light and happy.

You have achieved everything on your benefits form.

Imagine floating into that body in the future, and imagine, as best you can, what it's like.

This is what is called getting in touch with that end-state, or N-State energy.

- What does it look like?
- What does it sound like?
- What does it feel like?
- What does it taste like?
- What does it smell like?

Practice this technique every day, as often as you can. It

will change over time. You can do it instead of tools 8, or 9, or in addition to them.

How hypnosis helps:

Hypnosis can help the N-State experience feel so real that you can basically reach out and touch it. And when you get to that place, the N-State pulls you into the future. Little things are easier, and you begin to naturally move yourself in that direction because what you've done is just program your subconscious mind. You've given your SCM the roadmap, and set the course. That is where you're going.

Why it works:

We almost always do what we *feel*. So when you are connected with how you want to feel, you are much more likely to follow through on all the healthy habits you have set in place.

Scientifically, the reason this works is because you are activating the Reticular Activating System (RAS), which is basically a part of our brain that filters our experience. When you program your RAS with how you want to feel, your brain will be on the lookout for experiences that match what you've programmed it for. Your brain will basically be doing powerful pattern recognition based on your N-State to bring those experiences to you.

What this really means, is that the more you do this, and the more you are in touch with N-State, the faster you will get there because your daily experience – moment by moment – will be filtered to specifically direct you towards those experiences that match what you've asked for.

Laura's N-State

Here's an example of Laura's (from chapter 1) N-State:

What does it look like?

I'm happy. I can tell because I see a smile on my face, and I also look relaxed, and easy-going. I'm hiking with my family. The grandkids are there too – and we're having a great time being outside in this beautiful place together.

There's an ease of movement – I move with poise and grace, and it's just easy to walk around. There's a lightness in my step.

What does it sound like?

I hear sounds of laughter from my grandkids, and wind through the trees and gravel under my feet. I hear my grandson saying to me, "Nana, come find me!" as we play hide and seek and we're both laughing.

What does it feel like?

Adventurous, light, and free. I feel like I could do anything. I have a carefree attitude, and am open to new things. I'm not afraid anymore of doing physical things.

What does it taste like?

There's not much of a taste, maybe lemon water, or fresh and healthy.

What does it smell like?

The outdoors, with hints of the ocean.

After practicing her N-State for a few minutes each day,

Laura returned to my office the next week and we discussed her progress.

She mentioned that in the span of the week, she stopped at a park on the way home, and also went on a walk with her husband at the marina.

I asked her if she had done anything like that in a while, and she answered no – she hadn't. What likely occurred is that her N-State experience inspired her to have those experiences. Where she would normally just drive right by the park on the way home, this time she stopped there for 10 minutes. And where she would normally just run errands with her husband on the weekend, this time she made a special point to walk at the marina.

The N-State technique is extremely powerful, and the goal really is to *live in N-State at all times*. Imagine, if you felt happy, adventurous, light, and free from the inside (meaning the feelings are being generated by you using N-State), do you think it would be easier to stay on track and lose weight? Yes, of course it would. This is also why you've likely heard the phrase "Begin with the end in mind" – because it pulls you into that future. N-State will take you all the way there, and you can get better at it every time you practice it by making it more real.

The next chapter we move into phase 2 – Easy Weight Loss that is focused on optimizing the process to lose as much weight as possible week after week without feeling overwhelmed or deprived.

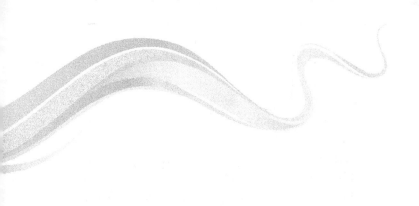

CHAPTER FIVE
Phase 2: Easy Weight Loss

There comes a point after phase one where people in the group are happy about their progress and the simplicity of the approach, and want to speed up their success with weight loss even more.

And it's common to want the process to speed up – to lose weight as fast as you can and make it to the finish line quickly. The problem with rapid weight loss though is that it's always associated with more work, and with deprivation. So rapid weight loss cannot be sustained. This is the problem with many diets; they are so restrictive that you can lose a bunch of weight on them initially, but the moment you're not able to follow the program anymore, the weight comes back.

It's like if I asked you to go the distance of one mile, on foot.

You could sprint it, yet by the end you could be exhausted and not be able to do anything else.

You could take your time, walk slowly, but you may get bored and get off track.

The best approach is to take it as quickly as you can, without pushing yourself. Meaning go as fast as you can without running or getting out of breath. That will enable you to *optimize* the distance for the long run.

And weight loss is the same. The goal is to find ways to accelerate weight loss for you, that don't also increase the work, stress, or energy involved.

That's what this chapter is about – **optimizing and accelerating weight loss.**

EAT HIGHER QUALITY FOODS

Easy weight loss includes doing things that are repeatable, and one of the primary elements is to really pay attention to the quality of the food you're eating. At this phase, you've already begun regular mindful eating, and now you're ready to take that to the next level.

Improving the quality of your food means you're getting more nutritionally dense food that does not increase inflammation, with fewer calories. This means you'll lose weight faster. Stick with wholesome, pesticide-, hormone-, and toxic-free food. Ideally locally grown. This often boils down to organic produce from your local grocer or farmer's market, and hormone-free meats.

It also means that mindful eating is becoming a habit – what we call unconscious competency. You're good at it, without thinking about it.

MOVING WITH MOMENTUM AND INTEGRATION

Easy movement is all about moving with momentum. Once you're consistently active for a few minutes each day, it's easy to continue the momentum by integrating movement into your daily life.

This is nothing new, I'm sure, but it's an important aspect of accelerated weight loss because it is *natural*. It is natural to start moving more – taking the stairs, walking at lunch, stretching throughout the day, once we have momentum – and the tools are geared around helping you integrate movement into your day.

FEELING BETTER: OPTIMAL ENERGY AND EMOTIONAL STATES

Once you're feeling better and losing weight, two areas to make weight loss repeatable include getting better sleep, and paying even more attention to how you're actually feeling.

When you're feeling good, and have enough energy because you had great sleep, it's easier to follow through on healthy habits.

The next chapter is all about tools to help make weight loss easy and repeatable.

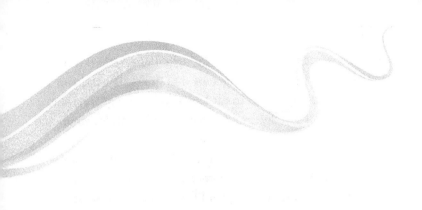

CHAPTER SIX

Phase 2: Tools to Make Weight Loss *Easy*

The tools in this section won't be applicable to everyone all the time; rather, they're intended to be used when needed.

Here's in general why they work: the brain doesn't want to change. It likes things to remain constant – even if that constant is uncomfortable, it's a known constant. So having a strategy for particular situations that includes a tool to use – a way to think about things, or an approach – means that you are much more likely to be successful.

These tools are ones that my clients have used for years – not always developed by me, by the way, but in many cases co-created out of necessity with clients.

The tools for ease of use – *easy* meaning effective, efficient, and repeatable – are really about tighter integration with your daily life. This means slight modifications to what you are doing that enable you to eat less (with higher quality), move more (in all you do), and feel better (with tools for emotional states and optimizing N-States).

This means the way to lose weight faster isn't just doing more of the same thing; rather it's integrating what you're doing into more areas of your life in ways that make sense.

TOOLS FOR EATING OPTIMALLY

Eating optimally is not eating perfectly. It's optimal for you. It's eating in a way that seamlessly fits into your lifestyle, and can be sustained.

11. LIVING IN THE GREY

Living in the Grey is a tool that is the opposite of black and white thinking – or the all or nothing approach. It's all about finding that proper balance between what you know is right for you (eating healthy or staying active), and the realities of daily living (eating out and being busy).

One of my recent workshop members had an experience that demonstrates this concept perfectly. Patricia was continuing to lose weight, but there was something that was holding her back. She loved Mexican food, and the last time she was there she was doing a good job of mindful eating

– until, that is, she had more than one margarita, which led to her eating more than she had planned.

She loved Mexican food, and this particular restaurant was her favorite place to enjoy time with her cousin. They had been going to lunch there for years and she didn't want to go anywhere else.

And this is where the Living in the Grey technique can be applied.

You don't have to eat perfectly to lose weight. Actually you can probably eat 80% relatively healthy food, and 20% not so great food, and still lose weight. As long as you're still eating only when you're actually hungry (tool #1).

Yet so many people have a hard time with stepping into that middle ground. They've been taught the "all or nothing" approach, or have struggled in the past. With some foods, like chips, cookies, or sweets, it is hard to step into that middle ground, so this technique cannot be used universally. But it's entirely possible with other situations, and eating out is one of those places.

I suggested to Patricia that she doesn't have to give up meeting her cousin for Mexican food. Then I asked if there was something else she *could* do to make eating there feel good to her, while she also enjoyed time with her cousin?

"Yes," she said "I would have been fine if I didn't have anything to drink. I'd still have fun, and very likely not overeat. "

After some hypnosis to lock in the change and get detailed insight, Patricia was happy with her new strategy for eating at the Mexican restaurant.

The key to this tool is that it is not rigid like an all-or-nothing approach – it's flexible. It's the flexibility inherent to this approach that makes it extremely valuable.

Patricia's Living in the Grey

Patricia returned a week later for the group session and reported that her experiment Living in the Grey worked wonderfully. She met her cousin at the Mexican restaurant, but she chose to have water instead of margaritas, and ate a healthy amount of food – not too much.

"I actually enjoyed it more than any time before – because I had fun, still enjoyed the food, but I didn't eat or drink too much so I didn't feel guilty later. It was perfect."

Ditch That Guilty Residue

Whenever we eat or drink something we know we shouldn't, it leaves a guilty residue that likely leads to eating more bad food.

Other examples of living in the grey include:

Being too busy to do your normal workout, so just do 1 minute instead.

Eating at a fast-food restaurant but having only a burger or sandwich – no fries or unhealthy drink. Note that eating at a fast food restaurant isn't a great idea because the food is typically not very high quality; however, sometimes things happen and we don't have another choice. For example, picking up kids at school, then driving to a game without having anything to eat and everyone is hungry. Yes, it would be better to have better planning, but living in the grey allows us to do something we know isn't the best choice, and make the most out of it.

How hypnosis helps:

Hypnosis is used to get to the root issue of why certain choices are made, or not made. It brings clarity to a situation so you can feel good about living in the grey, and making a choice that fits into your lifestyle. Sometimes it can be hard to go against what we've always been taught – and so if living in the grey feels uncomfortable to you, hypnosis can resolve that issue.

Why it works:

This technique works because it allows for flexibility. Anytime flexibility is introduced into a system – you win. When things are too rigid, then there's only one "right" answer, and if we don't get that right answer, then we feel guilty or bad that we failed. In the case of Patricia, there was no "right" answer. She wanted two separate things – to spend time with her cousin in a place they've always been to, and to continue eating healthy food. Was that her only choice? No, she could have suggested they eat somewhere else. That's also living in the grey – you have to find which works best for you and implement it in a way so it feels just right.

12. REDUCING SUGAR AND CARBOHYDRATES

It's important to talk about this technique, because there are a few really fantastic ways to reduce sugar and carbohydrates that

– using brain science and hypnosis – make getting off of these substances easier.

First the good news. Getting off sugar can reduce inflammation in the body in as little as a few days. This means, if you have joint pain, back pain, arthritis, or anything along those lines, and you know you eat too much sugar or carbs, you can expect to feel better.

I've had dozens of clients who report this to me, so although somewhat anecdotal, it's true in my experience. Get off the white stuff, and feel better in a few days. Your body will crave it, but after just a few days, the cravings will likely be gone.

If you're eating too much sugar – baked goods, candy, junk, that type of thing, that just needs to stop entirely. Cold Turkey usually. See tools for tea substitution (#14) and two bites (#15).

Here's how to do it, there are two approaches:

Reduce carbs by half across the board

The first approach is to reduce the carbohydrates in your life by half. This means if you have a cup of rice with dinner, have half a cup instead. If you also have a sandwich with lunch with 2 slices of bread, switch to a 1/2 sandwich with one slice of bread, and more fat or protein. Over time, continue to reduce it until it's the right amount for you – again usually around 25-50% of what you used to eat.

Reduce carbs to one serving per day

This approach is slightly different, instead of reducing carbs by half at each meal, you go down to only one serving of carbs per day at one meal, period.

This technique is usually harder, but it makes sense for some people, for example, if you eat healthy oatmeal for breakfast and want to continue with that, then you wouldn't have any carbs for lunch or dinner. That would be something like salad for lunch with healthy fat and protein, and vegetables and protein for dinner.

Both approaches work, but reducing carbs by half across the board is easier for most people.

How hypnosis helps:
Hypnosis helps by reinforcing the healthy change, and also by removing any resistance to a new style of eating.

Why it works:
It's clear from mounting evidence that moving away from a carbohydrate-based diet is the right approach for most people. Healthy fats and protein help keep us satiated, and provide lasting energy. You may be different, and if so, this technique is not for you.

13: EAT HIGH QUALITY FOOD

This technique is very straight forward and logical, yet it's often overlooked.

Imagine you have two piles of apples. One is grown locally without pesticides or other unnatural substances. The other is grown with pesticides, and travelled hundreds of miles to get to you.

The first apple will have a higher net energy and nutrition because your body will not have to discard any toxins.

The second apples will have a lower net energy and nutrition because of the toxins used in production your body has to now process out. But they both may have the same amount of calories. This means to get the same nutritional value, you'd have to eat more of the second apple, which means more calories.

In general, lower quality food leads to higher quantity, which means more calories for the same amount of nutritional value.

Eat higher quality food, and you'll naturally eat less.

How hypnosis helps:
If you have problems eating higher quality food, or prefer to eat foods that are of low quality because of taste or pleasure, hypnosis can help address those issues.

Why it works:
Your body is magnificent at giving you hunger signals based on need. When you eat higher quality food, you just need to eat less.

14: TEA SUBSTITUTION

Tea is a great substitution for food under many circumstances.

How it works:
Instead of something sweet after dinner, or an after lunch pick-me-up, have a cup of tea.

Why it works:
This technique works by the law of substitution. The brain doesn't actually want junk or snacks after dinner, it just wants something

pleasurable. And tea is an acceptable substitute for most people. Don't be confused thinking that a cup of tea will somehow seem like a bowl of ice cream – that's not how this works. It works by substitution. Of course, at first you may rather have the ice cream, but if you make yourself a cup of tea instead, after a moment of having the tea in hand, and enjoying the warmth and aroma, the ice cream more easily fades away. If you just try to quit ice cream cold turkey, the brain will continue to ask you for something – give you the idea of ice cream, or cookies, or something along those lines. When you give it a substitute, your brain has something else to focus on, and it's satisfied.

15: TWO BITES

Two Bites is a favorite technique in my first book, *Reprogram Your Weight*.

Two bites is a tool that is used when you want, or are expected or asked to eat something but you don't want to eat too much of it, (or you do very much want to eat too much of it, but you realize you'd feel guilty or bad later for doing so and would therefore wish to not have too much). For example, at your grandson's birthday party, if your grandson were to come up to you and ask if you were having birthday cake, you could politely employ the two bite approach, and have a piece of cake – then take only two bites.

Note that this technique doesn't work for every person, or every food. For some people, having one bite of their favorite foods makes it impossible to stop. That's a trigger food that needs to be eliminated from the diet entirely.

How hypnosis helps:

Hypnosis helps with this technique if you have problems thinking you'd be able to enjoy having only two bites. If the technique does not work, it can be an indicator that something deeper is going on. That the desire for pleasurable food is outweighing your body's other needs.

Why it works:

The law of diminishing returns is an economic term that can be applied here. It means that the first bite of something delicious is great. The second bite is good, but not as great as the first, and the third, even less spectacular. So by sticking to two bites of something, you're actually getting the best two bites, but without all the guilt that comes from eating the entire serving. This again brings flexibility into your toolbox for healthy eating that means it's easier to live your life, while still losing weight.

TOOLS TO MOVE MORE

16: DOUBLE UP: MOVE WHILE DOING SOMETHING ELSE

This technique is highly valuable, and many of my clients have used this as one of the catalysts to consistent and substantial weight loss.

Here's how it works:

Integrate being active into daily living by listening to music, podcasts, television, or anything else enjoyable while you exercise or do house work.

Moving More Can Be Easy

Most of my clients in group workshops are surprised by how easy it is to just move more once they start doing something else at the same time – listening to books on audio while walking and cleaning the house are both really successful approaches.

This technique is built in for actual housework – getting activity *while also* cleaning or gardening – and it's enhanced when you add something to it that makes it more interesting, like a book on tape or a podcast. This isn't for everyone – and for many clients they love gardening and would never dream of listening to anything while gardening, but for doing housework, they will. The chores don't seem so daunting if you're listening to a great song, or an interesting book, at the same time.

Why it works:

Integrating more activity into our daily lives helps build a new habit of just being more active. By adding some fun or interesting aspect to the work, now we have the brain that is interested in an otherwise boring or monotonous scenario, you're moving your body, and you're getting work done. It's a triple win.

17. PLAN ACTIVITY

One of the best ways to ensure that you are active every day – even if it's for one minute – is to know what you're going to do the night before.

Before you go to bed at night, know how you're going to be active the next day. Don't leave it up to chance.

Why it works:

If we don't plan for the important things in our life, it's very likely that they won't happen. Working out or staying active is one of those things that tends to get pushed out until later in the day, and then it just doesn't happen. Instead use the one minute of exercise (tool #7) along with knowing what you're going to do the night before to build in the consistency.

TOOLS TO FEEL GREAT

18. ELIMINATE NEGATIVE SELF-TALK

Science tells us that we're born with what is called a negativity bias. This means we are biologically programmed to focus on the negative for our survival.

The problem becomes when we experience significant levels of negative self-talk that keep us from being our best. If this is an issue for you, you likely already know it because you know what you say in your head to yourself is not very nice.

How it works:

Ask yourself, "Would I ever talk to a friend that way?" The answer is likely that you wouldn't and the reason is that it's not nice. But that's not the important part. The important part is that it doesn't work. If it did work, you wouldn't be reading this book.

So throw that old, outdated technique out, and instead do the following:

Talk to yourself like you would talk to a good friend going through the same situation. Tell her she's kind, and thoughtful. Focus on what is working and the positive aspects, and remind her that every day she can lose a little bit of weight, and feel lighter and better.

How hypnosis helps:

Negative self-talk is a protective mechanism that is out of control. Because it's biological and it usually happens in the privacy of our own mind, it can quickly get out of control for some people.

Note that the negative self-talk is often a learned behavior from a parent, teacher, or other authority figure. The talk itself can be in your own voice, or the voice of the parent, teacher, or authority figure.

If this is a problem for you, hypnosis can help make the switch to beneficial self-talk instead. Self-talk that is encouraging – is self-talk that actually will work to help you achieve your goals.

Why it works:

This biological construct is left-over from our caveman days, and although still useful in some situations – think crisis – we don't need it in our normal, non-crisis experiences. So a better technique is compassionate encouragement.

19. EMOTIONAL COMPASS AND METER

This technique is highly valuable, and one that can be used and improved upon over a lifetime.

The concept is that the direction is more important than the location. If you don't feel good, but you're moving toward better, that's great.

If you feel down, and moving toward worse, that's not great.

Here's what's important to understand about our emotional state: It's more likely to gradually move up or down the scale of feeling better or worse, and so reset an expectation to look for the direction (does that feel better?) rather than the exact location (I feel good, not great).

How hypnosis helps:

Hypnosis can help us to tap into that deeper feeling, and get accustomed to actually feeling and articulating what it is we're actually feeling. Some of this is related to emotional intelligence, or mastery, but some of it is also just using hypnosis as a tool to focus on what you're feeling, and then using that information to either switch direction, or validate you're moving in the correct direction.

Why it works:

So many people focus only on the location – meaning, I don't feel good, rather than which way they're heading – and when we do that, we can get discouraged. Know that emotional state and transformation is more like a scale, and moving from discouraged to hopeful is moving in the right direction. After hopeful you can feel encouraged, empowered, excited, and amazing.

Expecting to go from discouraged to amazing in one step is less likely to happen, so if that's what we expect, we'll often be disappointed, then feel even worse.

One way to think about this is to assign the best-feeling-state a number of 10. 10 represents the best feeling you can experience; some may call it joy, or love, or excitement. You get to determine what that means for you.

Then assign a number of one to the worst feeling you could have, which would be complete and total apathy – no desire to do anything at all. Even anger or frustration is a step above apathy.

Now at any point, even if you're at a one, do something to take you to a two. If you go for 10, you'll be disappointed and frustrated which will make it worse. Just get to the two, from there a three will be easy, and pretty soon you'll be at a four or five. And maybe a four or five is good for that day – it certainly feels better than a one. You don't always have to be up at a 10.

20. INCREMENTAL SUCCESS

Incremental success is a tool that focuses efforts on looking for small improvements. An example would be feeling good about walking for one minute every day for a week, and also knowing that next week you'll get better.

An alternative would be to be upset that you only walked one minute because in the past you used to run three miles a day. It's not helpful to feel discouraged – instead incremental success, recursive improvement, is a more likely approach.

Why it works

Incremental improvements are natural. A tree doesn't grow a new branch overnight – it grows a little every day. This allows for safe and healthy change, and it's the easiest way to make changes that last.

Putting It All Together

In this chapter we focused on tools to optimize weight loss and make it easy and repeatable. The ability to eat only when you're actually hungry gets easier over time, as you continue to get better with incremental success at everything you do. Integrating these techniques into your life is a way that begins to lead to everlasting results – which is what the next two chapters are all about.

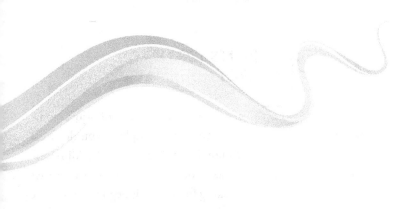

CHAPTER SEVEN:
Phase 3: Everlasting: Keep the Weight Off for Life

At this point in the group, clients are feeling great. They've lost weight in a way that seems simple – all they have to do is eat only when they're actually hungry, and find something else to generate good feelings. They're all accomplishing those two goals in unique ways that fit into their daily lives.

Yet, they also know they've lost weight before, and are hoping the good feelings and weight loss continue this time, so this next phase is all about how to keep the weight off for life. And in this phase, the techniques are focused on what actually works for the long-term – which is a consistent, yet flexible approach.

ONE OF THE BRAIN'S JOBS IS TO CONSERVE ENERGY

The brain conserves energy in a multitude of ways, some that we've already talked about. For example, if you don't eat when you're hungry the brain basically turns on the "dimmer" switch of your energy – aka your metabolism – because it's not getting the food it's asking for and so it begins to conserve energy. Your body does not need a continual stream of food like a lot of diet programs recommend; rather, just pay attention to when you're hungry and that's the best indicator.

The other way the brain conserves energy is by creating habits. Habits are pre-packaged executable programs that the brain creates to conserve energy. Through the process outlined in this book, and the corresponding hypnosis sessions, you will be reprogramming your habits so that they're in alignment with what you really want – which is to lose weight in a way that is natural, healthy, and sustainable for life.

Creating those healthy habits is a big part of permanent weight loss, and the best way to create these habits is consistency – but it's consistency with a twist – it's consistency with flexibility.

The best approach for long-term weight loss is to have a consistent, yet flexible approach. If you're consistent, but rigid, then the first time something stressful comes along in your life, or your normal routine changes, you'll get off track. This is what Laura was concerned about – that the holiday season would get her off track. And building in flexible consistency – finding that balance – is key. Here's how to do it.

FLEXIBLE CONSISTENCY

Flexible consistency includes *a variety of options to achieve the same result.*

The opposite of a variety of options is having a single way to achieve your result. This would be like only having one way to relax – for example, with food or alcohol. If you only have one way to relax, then you're very likely to use that one way over and over, with unwanted consequences.

Instead the best approach is to have multiple ways to relax, and given the three aspects we've discussed in this book, you'd want the following:

1. ***Multiple ways to eat mindfully.*** This means a variety of food, and options.
2. ***Multiple ways to move.*** Gardening, walking, taking the stairs, kayaking, cleaning your home. Not JUST the gym, or JUST the treadmill.
3. ***Multiple ways to feel good.*** Hypnosis, listening to music, crossword puzzles, sewing, pottery, dancing, singing.

When one of your ways is not available, or you become bored with it, then you switch to another option. Adding new options to your variety is an ongoing process, and it's actually fun and exciting for the brain to be on the lookout for new ways to move, eat mindfully, and feel good.

BALANCE AND MODERATION

Balance and moderation with what you do. This is about not over-doing it. Instead of working out really hard one day, then not being able to move the next, you're moderately active so you can do it again the next day. This can be hard because sometimes we're inspired to do more, but the goal really is to do things in such a way that you can also do them tomorrow.

DAILY IMPLEMENTATION

All three aspects should be done every single day. If a day goes by and you don't feel good, you may find yourself at the refrigerator in the evening looking for something to eat. Because you have not satisfied the brain's need for balance and homeostasis.

Keeping all of those things in mind, the best way to implement flexible consistency is to give your brain an expectation of success – to really know what that is like for you. Here's how it works.

MAXIMIZING N-STATE ENERGY

Have you ever felt excited about something, and that excitement fueled your entire existence for a period of time? One example of this is falling in love – in that state, everything is better. You're seeing the world through the eyes of love, basically, so when you look at a tree, the tree is more lovely. More beautiful. That is a state of mind, the state of being in love. And it's very powerful.

Tapping into N-State energy – how you want to be (look, feel, sound, smell, taste) once you're at your goal weight and achieved all other related goals – should be the same way. How do you know you're tapping into N-State energy? It should feel fun, and you'll be excited about it. It's something that you can work on and develop over time.

The point is that the N-State energy is self-generated. Now many will say that it's actually from spirit, or God, or you're tapping into Universal energy, but regardless of what you call it, it comes from within, and it's unlimited.

When you tap into that N-State energy, it will take you all the way to your desired end point.

Why N-State Energy is So Important

I want you to think about N-State energy as effortless. Think of someone you know that is at their ideal weight, but doesn't really have to try – they're not thinking about food all the time, or putting too much energy into shopping, weighing, or pointing their food. They're focused on other things.

And then think about the person who is just active. It's just part of their life. They're not trying to be active – they just are.

Permanent weight loss needs to be effortless – a combination of good strategy (mindful eating, moving, and feeling good), with the right habits (tools as described in this book). This doesn't mean there's zero effort, it means there's no struggle, and you can do it in a sustainable way.

N-State Eating

What's your relationship with food in that N-State? I recommend a loving relationship between food, your mind, and your body – you nourish your body with healthy, wholesome food when you're hungry, and it's also pleasurable. There is no residue of guilt or shame.

Create Your New Identity: what is your new identity regarding eating and food? Perhaps you used to be a "carb-oholoic," or someone with a "slow metabolism." And now it's important to change that to: You may identify with a person that just doesn't eat all that much, or someone who only eats when hungry. That is just who you are. You can enjoy food, but it's not the solution to every problem.

N-State Moving

How will you move your body in the N-State? Will you purposely work out every day, or do you want to integrate activity into your daily living with housework, gardening, and walking? Or do you want a more flexible approach – a balance of focused and purposeful activity, aka exercise, with some days when you're just busy and working your body through living?

Create Your New Identity: what is your new identity regarding moving your body? Are you an athlete, a walker, a hiker, or do you just identify with someone who likes to stay active and move through daily living? You may not love to be active, so perhaps you identify with the idea of just being healthy, and with the ability to go and do anything you want.

N-State Feeling

How will you feel in the N-State? Will you feel accomplished, peaceful, joyful, light? Who ARE you in this state? Are you a happy person, full of joy and peace? Are you focused, determined, compassionate?

Create Your New Identity: what is your new identity regarding how you feel? Instead of being stressed, or depressed, how about carefree? Or thoughtful? Or a renaissance-type of person who enjoys art and literature? You may consider being a compassionate caregiver who has something to share – perhaps your weight loss experience inspires you to help others do the same thing?

Knowing where you're going, and tapping into that N-State energy regularly, is one way to get that unlimited resource of passion and excitement that can take you all the way to your end goal.

Tapping into N-State is like jumping in the river and going downstream, instead of swimming against the current. Against the current is what most diet programs want us to do – go against our bodies' natural ways of doing things.

The next chapter is all about tools and techniques to capture the N-State energy to lose the weight and keep it off forever.

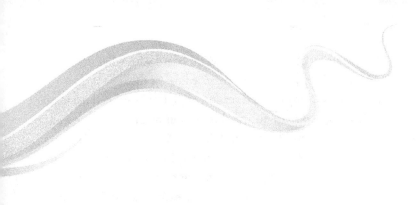

CHAPTER EIGHT

Phase 3: Tools to Keep the Weight Off for Life

The tools in this chapter will help you keep the weight off for life. They're more advanced tools that you'll use to integrate concepts of mindful eating, moving more, and feeling good into everyday living. You'll notice that some of the tools are not as directly related to eating or moving as in the previous two phases; rather, they're focused on helping you feel good about yourself, and they address common issues that my clients get tripped up by.

21. TOUCHSTONE OF N-STATE ENERGY

As described in the previous chapters, tapping into N-State energy gives you the ability to achieve your goals with minimal struggle by getting your SCM on board with what the plan is, then feeling excited and energized to get there.

This is an advanced version of tool #10 outlined in chapter 4. It's appropriate to use this version of the tool once you've had success in Phases 1 and 2.

This technique is all about using hypnosis to tap into that N-State energy, then creating a touchstone – an anchor or reminder of that state so it's easily accessible to you at any time.

Step 1: Complete the exercise in the previous chapter including the aspects of identity and who you want to be in regards to eating, moving, and feeling.

Step 2: Self-Hypnosis

Get in a comfortable position where you will remain undisturbed for at least 10 minutes. You can put on relaxing music if you'd like.

Note: Download the accompanying self-hypnosis audio recording at LighterBook.com.

Use your favorite self-hypnosis technique described in this book, including tool # 9 in chapter 3.

Step 3: Using what you wrote down in Step 1 as a guide, imagine yourself at your end-goal, at your ideal weight and having achieved all related goals. Make it as real as you can. Imagine that you *are that person.*

Step 4: Once you feel really good, and have a sense that you *are already becoming that person – you're just a younger version,* do the following:

Imagine, using the magic of the mind, that you are capturing that energy, that feeling, that knowing of who you are in that state and where you are heading. Capture it in your dominant hand and make a fist to lock it in really tight.

Next, move your hand up to your heart, and place it in your heart, knowing it will be there forever to guide and inspire you. To help you feel good, and know exactly what to do. Knowing it will change and grow over time, just like you will.

Step 5: When you're ready, emerge from hypnosis by simply counting from one up to three while you gently open your eyes.

You have created a touchstone.

Every time you want to feel good, touch your heart where you placed the N-state energy – it will come rushing back.

Every time you do feel good, touch your heart where you placed the N-state energy – it will reenergize it.

22. HIT THE RESET BUTTON

This tool is useful for many situations – especially under what I call "acute" feelings of anxiety, stress, or cravings. You are having a strong feeling (craving, stress, anger) that feels out of control and you want to eliminate it.

The benefit of this tool is it allows you to feel better in about 30 seconds. It's very powerful, and the more you use it, the more effective it becomes.

Here's how it works:

Whenever a situation comes up where you begin to feel out of control, stop. Awareness is the first step. Stop what you are doing and give yourself 2 minutes to complete the following:

1. Close your eyes to block out external distraction (make sure it's safe to do so).

2. Imagine squeezing the bad feeling (stress, anger, frustration, a craving for sweets) into your non-dominant hand. Squeeze as hard as you can without hurting yourself. Do this until it seems as if some of that negative feeling has dissipated.

3. Next, do what is technically called a "break-state" – think about something else entirely. For example, where's your favorite place to vacation? This is akin to a palate cleanser, except for your brain.

4. Next, imagine the N-State of this particular issue. What is the alternative option that you actually want? For example, if you're stressed, imagine feeling peaceful and serene. Imagine yourself floating peacefully through the water on a canoe, or listening to a gentle breeze as the sun goes down. If it's a craving, imagine feeling in control, and going on a walk instead (for example). Squeeze those good feelings into your dominant hand. Make it as real as you can.

5. Now, think again about the current situation and squeeze both hands powerfully and at the same time. This cancels the feeling out in your brain. It's neuroscience at work – you cannot have two competing thoughts at the exact same moment.

You should feel better, and the strong negative emotion will have dissipated. You can do this more than once if there's still a little of the negative emotion remaining.

How hypnosis helps

If you're struggling to imagine a powerful N-State for this situation, you can use hypnosis to get in touch with that feeling. The good feeling of what you want should always be more powerful than the one you don't.

Why it works

This technique works by cancelling out an automated response in our brain. Since you're associating two different outcomes and anchoring them to squeezing your hands, the brain doesn't know what to do when both hands are squeezed together. It's as if both states (the one you don't want, and the one you do) are triggered at the same time and the brain doesn't know which of them to follow. So they get cancelled out. The result is you feel instantly better; now you have a clear head and you can make a better choice – usually the one more in alignment with your N-State.

23. WORRY = ACTION

This simple tool can become a meme that will provide you years, maybe decades, of peace in return. And it's especially helpful if you tend to eat when you're stressed or nervous, because it can help eliminate stress eating entirely.

Here's how it works:

Worry is your conscious mind attempting to solve a problem. It's a good and noble thing to solve problems, I think.

However, many times our conscious mind gets off track and tries to solve problems that it actually can't solve – or doesn't have any control over to solve.

So this is what we want the conscious mind to know.

Worry = Action.

If there's action to take, it's a good thing to worry about it, notice what the action is, then take the action. Eating a cookie won't solve the problem. Eating ice cream won't solve the problem.

If there's no action to take, or it's not yours to fix, it's a waste of effort, time, and peace of mind to worry about it. *This does not mean you don't care! It simply means, it's not yours.*

If we worry about getting in a car accident on the freeway, we can put on our seat belt, and drive cautiously.

If instead we worry about another car hitting us, and all the possible cars on the road that could hit us at every turn, then when we drive we're anxious about all the things that could go wrong, we're more likely to cause our own accident. It can become a self-fulfilling prophecy.

Recognize that worrying about something you have no control over is really a waste of energy. It's inefficient. If you were doing something at work, and it didn't work – would you keep doing it? Ask yourself that: "Does this work, to worry about this thing?" If not, then stop it.

But Erika, you're thinking, if I could just not worry anymore by choosing not to, I wouldn't have to be here! Yes, I hear you, easier said than done.

Step 1: First, get conscious agreement that it doesn't make sense – logical sense, to worry about.

Once you can do that, move to the next step.

Note that sometimes you'll feel conflicted and you'll feel that mostly it isn't logical to worry about, but that there is one piece that is logical. In that case, break it down into its components. This is called chunking it down.

Take the parts that don't make sense to worry about, and they go in the illogical bucket.

Next take a close look at the remaining pieces – the ones that actually you can worry about because there's action you can take, then *take the necessary action.*

A feeling of internal conflict usually requires a bit of introspection and clarity, breaking down something large that we're conflicted about, into smaller pieces so they can be addressed one by one.

For example, in one of my groups a client was worried about her daughter travelling to a remote part of the world. This happened in the past, and she wasn't able to call her while she was there. As a result, she was up all night worrying about her being in danger. While she was worrying about her all night, she went back and forth to the kitchen – eating ice cream, cookies, and candy. She knew she was stress eating, but didn't know how to stop it.

Now her daughter was planning on travelling again and she didn't want the same thing to happen.

I asked her to break it down into parts. "Which part are you actually worried about?" I asked her.

She felt good about her daughter's travel plans because she researched them online, but she didn't like not being able to call her on the phone. That's the part that really made her nervous. If she could just get a phone call from her, she realized, she'd feel so much better.

Thankfully her daughter agreed to call twice a week, which alleviated a majority of the stress. She didn't stress eat, and she enjoyed the check-in calls from her daughter.

How hypnosis helps

If you're worrying or stressing too much over things that don't make sense, yet you're unable to resolve it using the above, hypnosis will reveal and release the root issue.

Why it works

The conscious mind wants to solve problems and be useful, but it's not the best tool for the job, just as a hammer isn't the best tool for every job. The process of identifying a strategy (worrying about what we can take action on), then chunking it down when there's conflict, is acceptable to the conscious mind's need for logic and control.

24. ONLY THINK ABOUT WHAT YOU DO WANT

This tool is an advanced technique applicable to every aspect of your life, and it's easy.

One principle of the mind is that whatever you focus on, grows. If I were to ask you right now to think about your toes, you'd become aware of them.

This principle of the mind is why it is so important to only think about what you *do* want to happen. This is important because it's natural to notice what is right now, and get stuck in that feeling. What I mean by that is you may feel the heaviness of your body, or that clothes fit too tight. And if you focused on those aspects, you'd likely feel bad. That feeling bad would likely lead to emotional eating.

Instead of thinking: I feel so heavy.

Think: I'm eating healthier and losing a little weight every day.

Instead of thinking: I don't want my jeans to be so tight.

Think: I've walked every day for a week and my jeans are getting a little looser.

Even if you've just started this plan, this technique still works:

Instead of thinking: I'm so tired of eating too much and feeling overweight and bad about myself.

Think: I'm trying something new that has worked for a lot of people. I like that I don't have to count calories or spend hours at the gym. It makes sense, and I'm hopeful.

Learning to think only about what you *do* want will help shift your thinking and **pull you towards** that end goal. If you're only thinking in terms of what you don't want, you'll pull yourself toward that!

Why it works:

This technique works because it's how our brain works – whatever we focus on, grows. So focus on what you do want, and you're much more likely to be successful.

25. ON SECOND THOUGHT: JUDGMENT

This tool is useful when you're wondering why you had a thought about a person or thing that you didn't want to have. Or felt bad about thinking something. The reason it's important is that in my groups, many clients have reported feeling bad about a having a judgmental thought, then later they'd overeat because of that bad feeling.

Realize that your first thought about a situation can be reactionary, and that you're not necessarily choosing it. For example, if you're walking down the street and you see someone talking loudly and behaving belligerently, a thought may pop in your head like "idiot," or "jerk."

And then you feel bad, because that's not who you are, you don't want to judge anyone. And so I want you to know that you're right, that's not who you are, not the real you. But it is how the primitive part of your brain is – you know, the part that's always trying to keep you safe. That type of reaction is a judgment based on a perceived and natural fear that is happening at the subconscious level.

So, here's how to resolve it.

Know that your first thought can be reactionary, and subconscious. It's usually driven by fear and intended to keep you safe. It's part of our negativity bias as discussed in tool #18.

You get to *choose your second thought.*

On Second Thought is a tool you apply when the judgment pops into your head: Just say to yourself, "On second thought, perhaps he's having a bad day and I wish him well." And you move on. Your second thought can be thoughtful, compassionate, or loving, or however you want it to be because you get to choose it.

Why it works:

As discussed in chapter 5, we have a negativity bias that is biological and designed to keep us safe. But we can consciously override that result with a second thought, which happens after the original thought. Preventing the original thought from arising in the first place is possible though, and that's where hypnosis can help resolve issues at the root level, and it can also be something you reprogram yourself to do over time.

When you apply this technique, you can continue feeling good about yourself and not end up emotionally eating later on in the day.

26. VALUES CONFLICT RESOLUTION

One of the things that keeps people from losing weight in the first place, is emotional eating – distracting themselves from feeling bad, by eating food. And one of the areas – that is so common for my clients to feel – is an internal conflict.

In my group, one of the members, Sue, had an internal conflict with her mom's passing. She was so happy her mom was no longer in pain, but she was also resentful and upset that she had to deal with it with no help from her siblings and now she's continuing to dealing with the issue because she's managing the estate. This feeling of conflict was preventing her from feeling good about thinking about her mom; she felt guilty because when she thought of her mom, she felt resentful and upset instead of loving, and because of this, she would turn to food to feel better.

You may have internal conflicts in your life as well, and many people don't know how to resolve them, so they ignore them or avoid dealing with them, so they get worse.

Here's a technique that helps to resolve these types of conflict.

- Step 1: Write down the conflicting parts, starting with how you feel.
- Step 2: Find the source of that feeling and this situation from a values perspective.
- Step 3: Bring the two parts together at a level that satisfies both parts.

Here's how it worked for Sue:

Feeling	**Value**
Peaceful	Well-Being
Resentful	Fairness

Sue felt peaceful for her mother because she values well-being, and her mother was suffering the last months of her life.

Sue felt resentful toward her family for not helping, and for her mother for not taking good enough care of herself so that she wouldn't need so much help near the end of her life.

Bringing these two together with hypnosis:

- **Step 1:** Use your favorite hypnosis technique in this book, and get into self-hypnosis.
- **Step 2:** Imagine both of these feelings and the value associated with each, and using the creative resources available during hypnosis, allow the mind to consider a solution to this conflict. The solution can be thought of as a *higher good.* It is above the conflict; this may not make sense to you now, but in hypnosis, your SCM will understand the meta message. Imagine the conflict as lower, and the solution as higher. This is also something that I work with my group participants on during our time together in class.

Sue imagined herself getting healthier. She saw herself losing weight, and not burdening her own family with her health issues. She also saw herself *taking care of her own end of life issues*, she planned on making arrangements to review her will and end of life process with her lawyer and family, and on ensuring her kids wouldn't have to go through what she was put through.

Why it works:

We can't go back in time and fix things, but residual emotional states of conflict always have some higher purpose, some meaning, and when we know how to get that information, the conflict is resolved and the emotion is transformed to a better feeling emotion – we feel better.

In the end, Sue felt a sense of peace regarding her mother's passing, and she took care of her own estate and was even more inspired to continue losing weight. She didn't feel bad anymore about her mom's passing, so she wasn't emotionally eating. She also delegated work to her siblings to share some of the burden regarding the mom's estate, and if they didn't want to help, then they wouldn't receive a fair benefit either. She felt good about that, and it made sense to her heart and mind.

27. REDUCE OVERWHELM WITH NEXT, SMALLEST THING

Have you ever taken too big of a bite of food? That's exactly what I want you to think of the moment you feel overwhelmed, because that's all overwhelm is – you have taken too big of a bite of whatever it is you're thinking about.

This is an important and common issue to address because in my experience, almost all of my group participants feel overwhelmed about a situation in their life and it causes significant stress. It could be at work, with family, or just trying to clean out the garage.

Feeling overwhelmed often leads to an inability to get started. People feel stuck, and that feels bad and leads to emotional eating.

Here's how to fix it:
- **Step 1:** Imagine yourself taking too big of a bite of

food – for me, it's an apple. My picture in my head is me with an apple in my hand, half gone, and the other half in my mouth.

- **Step 2:** Take a deep breath
- **Step 3:** Laugh. It's going to be just fine. It's just too big of a bite.
- **Step 4:** Take a smaller bite: what's the *next, smallest step* you can take?

This is so important. Every big project, every large goal, is made up of small steps.

It could be a smaller part of whatever you are thinking of, or not thinking so far in the future.

How hypnosis helps:

Hypnosis can help alleviate the stress of feeling overwhelmed by identifying the underlying root issue causing stress. It can also help align you with the higher purpose for the sense of overwhelm, and connect you with the new strategy of the next, smallest step.

Why it works:

This technique works by giving your conscious mind guidance on how to address issues in our life that really are too big for us to consume all at once. The result is you're able to get things done, and not overeat.

28. THE POWER OF SURRENDER

Have you ever been trying to remember something, only to think of it while doing the dishes, gardening, or in the shower?

Why does that happen?

What about the expression, "I'll sleep on it," does that really work?

The answer to both, is surrender. **Surrender of the Conscious Mind**.

You likely have a definition of surrender already in your head, and so I want you to know the definition of surrender in this case is very different.

The CM really wants to be the boss of everything. Think of your CM as a control freak, so every single little thing that comes into your head and heart, your CM wants to be in charge of.

And the CM is *not* the best tool for the job in many cases because whatever you're thinking or worrying about is bigger than the 7-9 bits of information that your CM can handle.

So as long as your CM is trying to fix the problem – hint: as long as you are consciously focused on thinking about it – your SCM is blocked from providing the answer.

This tool is important because for big issues in our life – like should I change careers, or how to address a delicate situation with a loved one – the conscious mind is not very good at finding an appropriate answer. So we can feel stuck, and that stuck feeling – not knowing what to do, or feeling helpless – can lead to overeating.

Here's how it works:

- **Step 1:** Notice that you're trying to figure something out consciously, yet it's not working. You're not getting the answer that way.
- **Step 2:** Stop focusing on finding the solution by specifically doing something. Something with your hands that is easy to do tends to work best, for example: dishes, shower, gardening, crafts. Sleep works as well, but that of course can take more time.
- **Step 3:** Eventually, you will have a lightbulb moment.
- **Step 4:** Tell your CM and SCM thank you, and feel really awesome. You just learned how to optimize your own brain and thinking, and found a new way to avoid emotional eating.

How hypnosis helps:

Hypnosis is basically getting the CM to take a short vacation so we get direct access to the SCM the entire time. Sometimes the CM tries to check in during mid-vacation, but with practice, the CM will recognize the value of a short vacation, and it will look forward to the break from being the boss at all times.

Why it works:

By focusing your CM on something else to do, the SCM has an opportunity to provide you the answer.

29. CATCHING THE SUNRISE

This technique was inspired by a client, and my trip to Maui. It's important because it can help you to stop emotionally eating when you have a bad situation in your life that you feel you can't get out of or change.

This story was shared by one of my group participants, Amy. Amy was stuck in a bad situation at home. She didn't love her husband anymore, and he didn't love her either. They both agreed to this, but she had 2 young kids and wanted to stay together for them. Her own parents had divorced at a young age, and her younger brother never got over their divorce. According to her, it ruined his life. He felt insecure, and unhappy, and to this day he hasn't bounced back. He's 41 years old. She did not want that to happen to her kids if they got divorced.

Setting aside the other options that Amy has, and whether or not you agree with her and her husband's choice – she's in a bad situation and she's making a choice. She's choosing to stay in one bad situation because in her mind, it's better than the only other perceivable option.

It reminded me of a trip to Maui where I wanted to catch the sunrise at Mt. Haleakala. The views were supposed to be spectacular, and so I signed up for the trip. The only problem is that it meant leaving the hotel around 1:15. In the morning. That's right, it meant leaving at 1:15 AM. Right in the middle of my night and day.

So this technique is all about making whatever choice you make – whatever you're going through – *worth it*.

For Amy, if she's going to choose to stay at home with a husband she doesn't love, but with kids she does, she needs to make it *worth that choice*.

How to do it:

If you're stuck somehow in a situation that seems terrible, or unmanageable, make it worth it by enjoying other aspects of your life. Meaning if you're stuck in a job you hate, make it worth it by having the time of your life in the evening.

If you're stuck in a marriage that's hard, make everything outside that time of your life worth it.

Don't drag your crappy job home with you at night. It's bad enough you're still there. Leave it there.

Don't drag your bad relationship around with you at other times. Amy is choosing to stay in a bad relationship for her kids, but if she lets the bad relationship ruin her entire life, she is not doing her kids any good. So she made it worth it. She learned to go out of her way to ensure time with her kids is amazing, and what she found was that when she focused on what she wanted – that end result – then her relationship with her husband improved as well.

A big part of how to do this is to focus your mind on something else when you're not at the job, or with the person. Specifically think of something else, and focus on making the rest of your life amazing. Or use one of the techniques in this book to reduce the feeling bad – like #21 Touchstone of N-State Energy, or #22 Hit the Reset Button. Both of those can help to change how you're thinking and feeling in the moment.

How hypnosis helps:

Hypnosis is really helpful when making hard decisions about things in your life like this – it can help to bring clarity to tough decisions so the right one can be made. And if the choice is to stick with one bad situation to avoid another (no judgment), then stick with that decision and make it worth it.

What I see instead, is someone stuck in a bad relationship that they don't feel they can realistically get out of (whether it's with a person or job), and then they also let that relationship ruin the rest of their life as well.

Why it works:

Focusing the mind on other things that make you happy will alleviate the stress of a challenging situation. Remember – you can't purposefully stop thinking of something, you have to specifically think of something else instead.

30. HELP – IT'S NOT WORKING!

Sometimes clients call me for a "booster" session and say I'm stuck! Or something happened and I'm not losing weight anymore!

Breathe. It's going to be just fine.

There's usually two reasons for this:

1. Something new and unexpected has come up, and it's easier for them to get additional support to work through it quickly.

Or

1. They've stopped doing what was working. They just stopped doing it.

This is usually resolved by the following: re-read the book and get back on track. Ask yourself the following:

1. Am I eating only when hungry? Note this is the number one reason people come back to see me; they stop doing this for a variety of reasons.
2. Am I moving my body?
3. Am I getting some relaxation and enjoyment every day? Am I generating those good feelings?

If the answer is no to any three of the above, you'll likely be feeling off track, and weight loss will stall, or you'll move in the wrong direction.

Hypnosis is not magic. I wish it could be so that I could promise my clients permanent weight loss, but the reality is you have to keep doing the techniques and applying the strategy. Hypnosis is what we work on in group sessions. It helps by making adoption of the tools easy and eliminating the root cause, and since they're natural and healthy, there's usually little if any resistance to doing them other than natural resistance to change.

Sometimes we just forget.

Have you ever forgot something really important?

Me too. It's OK.

Call a compassionate hypnotist, re-read the book, watch a video. Do what worked for you last time. You'll get back on track.

If you can't figure it out consciously – that's a sign that

whatever it is, is subconscious, so see your hypnotist to figure it out.

Putting It All Together

There is one technique left – the 31st, and it's how to put all of it together into your life. The next chapter brings the entire process full circle for you to lose weight and keep it off for the rest of your life.

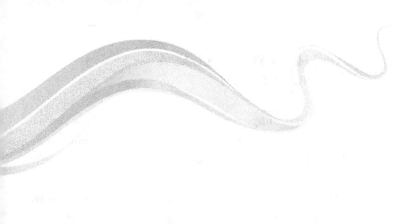

CHAPTER NINE
The Most Important Thing

Once again, I want you to imagine yourself now closer to that N-State, your end goal. Since you picked up and started reading this book, you're even further along your path. It's not only about weight loss, it's about feeling lighter in your body, mind, and heart. It's waking up in the morning feeling energized and refreshed. It's having something to look forward to every day, it's taking food off the pedestal and putting it where it belongs – there for energy and nutrition. It's a life where you do things daily that feel good, and generate those feel-good feelings.

The undercurrent supporting all of this work is one technique – one tool that is the most important of all, and it's recognizing how you feel.

31. USE HOW YOU FEEL AS A GUIDANCE SYSTEM

This is the most important thing to remember – how you are feeling tends to drive your behavior, and if you're not feeling well, food won't solve the issue unless it's because you're hungry!

This technique is so important it can take a lifetime to master – but you can get better at it every day. Here's how it works:

1. Notice how you're feeling, and address it properly:
    * If you're hungry, eat something healthy.
    * If you're tired, rest or listen to a hypnosis or relax-ation recording to recharge or energize yourself.
    * If you're bored, do something to challenge yourself.
    * If you're feeling other emotions – like anger, sadness, or loneliness, do something to address those issues. Eating will not solve them. If you don't know how to fix them or they're unresolv-able, do something else.
2. Over time, your "new normal" will be more relaxed, and peaceful than ever before.
3. That's the goal, for your new normal to be relaxed, peaceful, and fun. That will be the default for you.
4. Once your new normal is more relaxed, peaceful, and fun, it's even easier to notice when things aren't going well.

Once you're feeling better in general, and are experiencing more moments of peace and enjoyment in your life, it's even easier to notice when you're not feeling well – and adjust things before they get out of control.

And that's exactly what my clients do in group sessions.

They begin to experience a "new normal" in life that is happier and more peaceful. They don't think about food nearly as much, and eat only when they're actually hungry.

Group participants tend to lose weight every week and in our last session together share their stories of transformation.

Here's one story from a group participant, Jennifer, that I'll never forget.

Jennifer shared that she felt free of the weight-loss struggle. She knew she could lose weight week after week by eating only when she was actually hungry, then doing those things in her life that generated the good feelings. She didn't use food anymore to create the happiness in her life, nor was it the sole provider of joy. Instead she was drawing, and doing pottery again.

"I think I can do this on my own now," Jennifer said. "I wake up in the morning and I'm not depressed about myself, or my issues with my body or food. I know it will take time for me to lose all the weight, but the struggle is gone. Now I know all I need to do is eat only when I'm hungry, and my body takes care of the rest. It's such a relief."

When she doesn't feel well, meaning she's sad, stressed, or bored, she does something to address those feelings. She listens to music, or goes on a walk. Those things actually do help her to feel better.

"Now I just pay attention to how I'm feeling – whether it's an emotional feeling like boredom, or a physical feeling like hunger or needing to rest or de-stress. When I take care of myself, I'm a better mom, wife, and employee. It makes me happy to know that I'm in charge of that part, and also realizing that no one else is! No one else really can make me happy, and I can't make anyone else happy either. All I can do for my son is continue to support and love him, it's not worth me being miserable worrying about him or my parents – I can't do anything about that. Instead now I focus on what *can* be done – and that's me taking care of me, a little each day, paying attention to how I'm feeling and addressing it. I can do this. A weight has been lifted from my heart, my shoulders, and from my body as well. Thank you, Erika."

And so here is my wish for you:

That every day you wake knowing that you're enough. You are lovable, and good. You awake feeling rested, and with something to look forward to in the day. You have energy and desire to do what it is you want to do, and nothing stops you. You eat only when you're actually hungry, and anytime you get an idea for food but realize you're not hungry, you just know that it's your brain trying to get your attention – so listen. What is it you really need? Is it a break from what you're doing? Then rest, or listen to music. Is it to de-stress? Are you bored? Challenge your brain with something else to do. This gives you control back. And when you're paying attention to how you're feeling on a small scale – before it gets out of control – then you realize you really are in control of how you feel – you're in control of the response. This sets you free.

I know with the right combination of these tools integrated into your life, you will be successful. I see it every day in the hypnosis office and classroom. It's powerful to feel in control of eating again, then losing weight and finally feeling like your life is headed in a direction that in general brings daily happiness. Not happiness that comes from a box of cookies or a bag of chips, but genuine, internal happiness. It's finding true joy and fulfillment from deep within that enables us to return to a healthy weight and stay there for life, and I realize that working with so many clients throughout the years has really been about helping them find that light within them – what brings them true happiness and joy. Happiness generated from within. It's the singing, the dancing, the pottery – hiking, being in nature, spending time with people you love, adventures, helping others, growing spiritually, and feeling more alive. That is my wish for you and I know for certain it is achievable. I see it and am honored to be a part of it every day. I can't wait to help you get started re-igniting the light within you. Feeling lighter, happier, and more peaceful every day of your life and bringing that genuine love and lightness to everyone in your world.

With all my love,

Erika

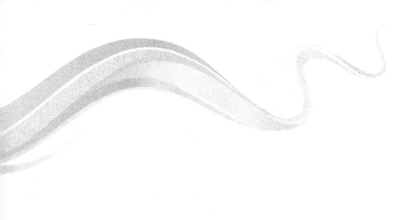

Acknowledgements and Resources

To each of my clients, I am forever grateful for your willingness to share what is working for you so that others can benefit, for your generosity of spirit, and for showing up willing and ready to release whatever is holding you back.

To my loving and supportive family and friends and colleagues, thank you for your ongoing love and support while writing this book.

To everyone at the Author Incubator, including Angela Lauria and Cynthia Kane, thank you for helping me find a way to share my work and help others with the message.

To the Morgan James Publishing team: Special thanks to David Hancock, CEO & Founder for believing in me and my message. To my Author Relations Manager, Bonnie Rauch, thanks for making the process seamless and easy. Many more thanks to everyone else, but especially Jim Howard, Bethany Marshall, and Nickcole Watkins.

HYPNOSIS TECHNIQUES IN THIS BOOK

Many of the tools in this book I've learned from working with hundreds of clients over many years. They were born out of necessity and through a collaboration between me and my clients in private and group sessions. When clients have success in a situation, I notice the how and why it works, then turn it into a reusable technique for other clients to capitalize on. This is a clear benefit of focusing on helping so many people lose weight with hypnosis.

Other tools detailed in this book are a synthesis of some of the most advanced and powerful hypnosis techniques used in the profession that I've learned from other hypnotists and teachers.

I've taken these techniques and applied them to the issue of weight loss in a systematic way that has enabled my groups and clients to consistently lose weight week after week and keep it off in a way that is easy for them – without the struggle.

Thank you to all of my colleagues, trainers, and teachers for all that you do, and especially to the following hypnotists whose techniques I've incorporated in whole, or in part, into this book and program:

Calvin D. Banyan

- Cal Banyan, the creator of 5-PATH ® and 7th Path Self-Hypnosis ® was and remains instrumental in my understanding and application of hypnosis.

- Chapter 2, Why Hypnosis
- Chapter 9, #31: Use How You Feel as a Guidance System

Melissa Tiers
- Chapter 8, #27: Reduce Overwhelm and Next, Smallest Thing

John Overdurf
- Chapter 4, #10: N-State (End-State)

Don Mottin
- Chapter 3, 1 Minute of Activity

Richard Bandler
- Chapter 8, #22 Hit the Reset Button and #26 Values Conflict Resolution

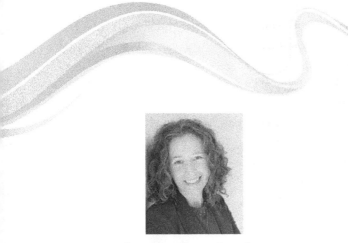

About the Author

ERIKA FLINT is an award-winning hypnotist, best-selling author, speaker, and a co-host of the popular podcast series *Hypnosis, Etc.* She is the founder of Cascade Hypnosis Center in Bellingham, WA, and the creator of the **Reprogram Your Weight** system of lasting weight loss without the struggle.

Before becoming a hypnotist, Erika designed software for the high-tech industry. She was working in that field for over a decade when she realized how interested she was in the most powerful computing device available – the human mind. Now she combines her analytical expertise along with powerful hypnosis techniques and her compassion for people to help clients utilize their most powerful asset – their mind.

She has assisted hundreds of clients with weight loss by

helping them reprogram how they think and feel. Her unique design and approach helps clients tap into their own inherent power and keep the weight off once and for all.

Erika's heartfelt approach is the trademark of her work. She values authentic connections with people and works to reveal the wonderment at the core of each individual.

She lives in Bellingham, WA, with her family including three sweet cats and a happy rescue dog who looks like an ewok and loves to play soccer.

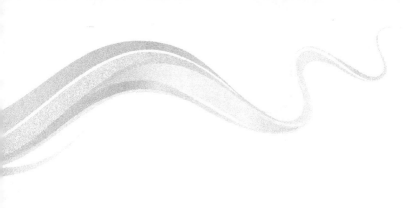

Thank You

Thank you for reading this book. It's my great honor and pleasure to share these tools and techniques with you.

For even faster results, make sure to use the hypnosis recordings and other material that accompany this book located online here:

www.LighterBook.com/hypnosis-recordings

For additional support including group and personal programs, visit www.**LighterBook.com.**

With much love,
Erika Flint

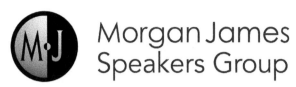
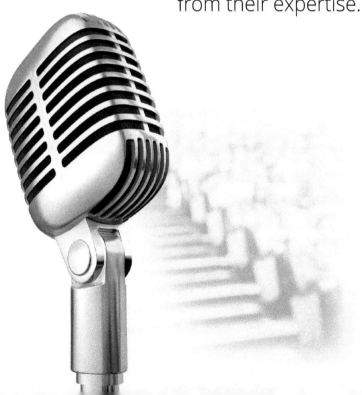

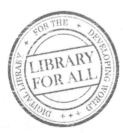 Morgan James makes all of our titles available through the Library for All Charity Organization.

www.LibraryForAll.org